Clinical Care
of the
Terminal Cancer
Patient

Clinical Care of the Terminal Cancer Patient

BARRIE R. CASSILETH
*Director, Division of Human Resources, University of
Pennsylvania Cancer Center*
*Research Assistant Professor of Medicine, University of
Pennsylvania School of Medicine*

PETER A. CASSILETH
*Professor of Medicine, University of Pennsylvania School of
Medicine*
*Associate Chief, Hematology–Oncology Section, Hospital of the
University of Pennsylvania*

Lea & Febiger · *1982* · *Philadelphia*

Lea & Febiger
600 Washington Square
Philadelphia, Pa. 19106
U.S.A.

Library of Congress Cataloging in Publication Data
Main entry under title:

Clinical care of the terminal cancer patient.

Bibliography: p.
Includes index.
1. Cancer—Treatment.   2. Terminal care.
I. Cassileth, Barrie R. II. Cassileth, Peter A.
[DNLM: 1. Neoplasms—Therapy. 2. Terminal care.
QZ 266 C6413]
RC270.8.C54   616.99'4029   82-15222
ISBN 0-8121-0854-X   AACR2

Cover photograph and design by E. F. Beasley
Copyright © 1982

Production Assistant, S. H. Davis

Flowers kindly donated by Lawrence Joas
ATCO Greenhouses, Atco, New Jersey

PRINTED IN THE UNITED STATES OF AMERICA

Print Number   3   2   1

To our children:
Jodi, Wendy, Gregory, and David, with our love and
respect for their patience and understanding.

Preface

Certainly we must rage, rage against the dying of the light, fighting with every tool at our disposal. But when therapeutic interventions fail and the patient draws inevitably into that good night, "do not go gentle"* becomes the inspiration no longer for the struggle to prolong life, but rather for the task of assistance in the face of certain death. And the effort here, requiring creativity, clinical skills, compassion and judgment, is no less difficult or worthy. The call now is not for retreat but its opposite—for the courage to remain with the dying though bereft of our standard armor and usual goal: therapy aimed at cure.

The responsibilities and obligations of the clinician do not end when physical disease eludes cure. There is more to be done, more needed by the patient, more that the clinician has to offer. But it is difficult terrain for those schooled in active intervention toward eradication of disease, and it is easy to feel defeated as a result of our inability to block approaching death. There is such a thing as a good death, just as there is a good life. In both instances the measure is relative and subjective; in both instances useful, beneficial intervention on the part of caregivers stems from skills that can be learned.

These skills encompass a broad range of therapies and capacity: knowledge of appropriate diagnostic and palliative techniques; interpersonal skills; and the ability to determine if, when, and how to intervene on the patient's behalf in any sphere. We have ap-

---

*Dylan Thomas: "Do Not Go Gentle Into That Good Night." Collected Poems, 1953.

proached the problem of care of the terminal cancer patient from diverse perspectives in order to cover its manifold issues and implications. Some issues are approached from more than one vantage point. Pain, for example, is covered in separate chapters on its clinical manifestations, its psychophysiology, and its specific control.

This book is aimed at oncologists and other clinicians who confront the demands of terminal malignant disease with their patients, and who strive to meet the physical and psychosocial challenges that such patients represent.

We gratefully acknowledge the willing efforts of the contributors, and the dedication and skill of Ms. Susan H. Davis in the preparation of the manuscript.

Philadelphia   Barrie R. Cassileth
                                                    Peter A. Cassileth

Contributors

Janet L. Abrahm, M.D.
   Assistant Professor of Medicine, Hematology–Oncology Section, University
   of Pennsylvania School of Medicine

Barrie R. Cassileth, Ph.D.
   Director, Division of Human Resources, University of Pennsylvania Cancer
   Center
   Research Assistant Professor of Medicine, University of Pennsylvania School
   of Medicine

Peter A. Cassileth, M.D.
   Professor of Medicine, University of Pennsylvania School of Medicine
   Associate Chief, Hematology–Oncology Section, Hospital of the University
   of Pennsylvania

Lon O. Crosby, Ph.D.
   Research Assistant Professor of Nutrition in Surgery, University of
   Pennsylvania School of Medicine
   Executive Director, Clinical Nutrition Center, Hospital of the University of
   Pennsylvania

Judy A. Donovan, R.N., M.S.
   Nurse Coordinator, University of Pennsylvania Palliative Care Program

Arnold Feldman, M.D.
   Associate Clinical Professor of Psychiatry, University of Pennsylvania
   School of Medicine
   Director of Liaison Consultation Psychiatry, Pennsylvania Hospital
   Psychiatric Consultant, Hospice Program, Pennsylvania Hospital

Tovia G. Freedman, M.S.W., A.C.S.W.
   Family Therapist, University of Pennsylvania Palliative Care Program

John H. Glick, M.D.
   Associate Professor of Medicine, Hematology–Oncology Section, University
   of Pennsylvania School of Medicine
   Director, Division of Clinical Research, University of Pennsylvania Cancer
   Center

Michael H. Levy, M.D., Ph.D.
Adjunct Assistant Professor of Medicine, University of Pennsylvania School
  of Medicine
Director, Palliative Care Service, Fox Chase Cancer Center
Chief, Lung Cancer Section, Department of Medicine, Fox Chase Cancer
  Center

Peter C. Nowell, M.D.
Professor of Pathology and Laboratory Medicine, University of Pennsylvania
  School of Medicine
Associate Director, University of Pennsylvania Cancer Center

Joanne Packer-Weiss, R.N.
Discharge Planning Coordinator, Department of Nursing, Hospital of the
  University of Pennsylvania

The Reverend John B. Pumphrey, B.A., M.Div.
Director, Department of Pastoral Care, Hospital of the University of
  Pennsylvania
Chaplain, Episcopal Community Services, Philadelphia

Melvyn P. Richter, M.D.
Assistant Professor of Radiation Therapy, University of Pennsylvania School
  of Medicine
Director, Department of Radiation Therapy, American Oncologic Hospital

Arnold J. Rosoff, J.D.
Associate Chairman and Associate Professor of Legal Studies, and Associate
  Professor of Health Care Systems, Wharton School, University of
  Pennsylvania

Gerard A. Ruch, Ph.D.
Assistant Professor of Pharmacology, University of Pennsylvania School of
  Medicine

Edward L. Schieffelin, Ph.D.
Senior Research Fellow, Institute for the Study of Human Issues,
  Philadelphia

Donald H. Silberberg, M.D.
Professor and Chairman, Department of Neurology, University of
  Pennsylvania School of Medicine

James L. Stinnett, M.D.
Associate Professor of Psychiatry, University of Pennsylvania School of
  Medicine
Director, Psychiatric Consultation-Liaison Services, Hospital of the
  University of Pennsylvania

Contents

Chapter 1

Tumor Biology: Evolution Toward Terminal Illness

Peter C. Nowell

Not all tumors evolve to a clinically terminal stage. Some remain benign and localized; some are treated early and cured; and other early tumors may be destroyed by the body's immune system before they attain metastatic capacity. This chapter focuses on the emergence and evolution of cells that do attain the ability to invade and to metastasize, leading to a fatal outcome. The discussion that follows establishes a theoretic framework which helps to explain, at a cellular level, how cancers arise. Although this exposition is conceptual, it is based on extensive experimental data derived from studies of tumors in animals and in humans.

The model below (Fig. 1–1), a representation of tumor evolution, serves as a basis for discussion.

The model has two basic underlying tenets. First, *most tumors begin from a single cell.* A normal cell (T_1) undergoes a heritable change for one or more of a variety of reasons, discussed later, which alters the cell permanently so that it no longer responds normally to growth regulation. As it begins to divide, the altered cell, T_1, and its progeny have a selective growth advantage over normal, adjacent cells. The exact nature of the selective advantage is unknown, but because the cellular alteration is heritable, the cell's progeny also are characterized by the same selective growth advantage. This population of cells (T_1) begins to expand at the expense of normal cells in the area, forming an early tumor. A neoplasm, therefore, may be defined as a clone—a population of

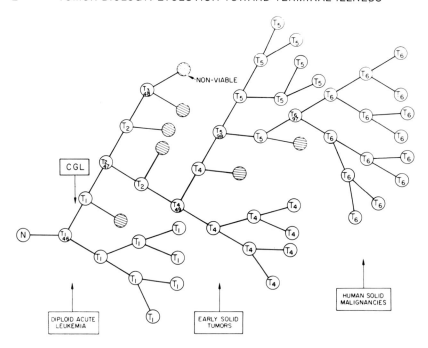

Fig. 1–1. Model of clonal evolution in neoplasia. Carcinogen-induced change in progenitor normal cell (N) produces a diploid tumor cell (T_1, 46 chromosomes) with growth advantage permitting clonal expansion to begin. Genetic instability of T_1 cells leads to production of variants (illustrated by changes in chromosome number, T_2 to T_6). Most variants die, due to metabolic or immunologic disadvantage (hatched circles); occasionally one has an additional selective advantage (for example, T_2, 47 chromosomes), and its progeny become the predominant subpopulation until an even more favorable variant appears (for example, T_4). The stepwise sequence in each tumor differs (being partially determined by environmental pressures on selection), and results in a different, aneuploid karyotype predominating in each fully developed malignancy (T_6). Earlier subpopulations (for example, T_1, T_4, T_5) may persist sufficiently to contribute to heterogeneity within the advanced tumor. Biologic characteristics of tumor progression (for example, morphologic and metabolic loss of differentiation, invasion and metastasis, resistance to therapy) parallel the stages of genetic evolution. Human tumors with minimal chromosome change (diploid acute leukemia, chronic granulocytic leukemia) are considered to be early in clonal evolution; human solid cancers, typically highly aneuploid, are viewed as late in the developmental process. (From Becker, F. (ed.): Cancer: A Comprehensive Treatise. Vol. I. 2nd Ed. New York, Plenum, 1981.)

cells arising from a single cell—comprised of cells with an acquired, heritable selective growth advantage and lacking normal responsiveness to local growth regulation.

The second tenet of this model (Fig. 1–1) is that a degree of *genetic instability exists in this population of cells.* Every time one of these cells divides, there is increased probability for further genetic alteration within the population as compared to normal cells. The initial alteration that confers the heritable growth advantage on the cell can be considered an acquired mutation. As this population divides, the likelihood for further mutation increases because of the system's instability. Mutations that occur subsequently result most frequently in a selective disadvantage for the cell, or at least in no additional advantage. Most of these mutations will not become apparent within the population or, if they are detrimental, the cells will die. Occasionally, however, an additional mutation occurs yielding an additional selective growth advantage not only over normal cells, but over the initial neoplastic population as well.

The ensuing new subpopulation (T_2) grows and, ultimately, overgrows the original tumor. Because of the genetic instability of the system, there is, over time, a tendency for increasing degrees of genetic variation. Sequentially, additional subpopulations are generated. These are incrementally more abnormal genetically; and they are selected increasingly for those characteristics associated with malignancy.

The diagram shown in Figure 1–1 indicates only six sequential populations of cells with serial mutations. For most of the common cancers of man, these mutations—some successful in terms of tumor growth and others not—may occur over many more steps before tumors are detectable clinically. When clinical diagnosis becomes possible, the tumor is far removed not only from the normal cell (N), but also from the initial cell that first acquired neoplastic characteristics (T_1).

The sequence of events described above reflects chance mutation and the selective pressures that exist in a given tumor. Although the particular sequence may not be completely random, it does exhibit variability. The selective pressures allowing a particular mutant to grow certainly differ from tumor to tumor (breast cancer versus lung cancer, for example), and from patient to patient. Thus, breast cancers in two patients may appear identical, but because they have evolved differently biologically, they may well behave differently on a clinical basis in terms of rate of growth, spread, and response to treatment.

The sequential alterations are cumulative. They produce a population that increasingly deviates from normal over time, and that becomes more and more malignant and aggressive. This is a phenomenon that is recognized clinically and biologically as "tumor progression."

The probability of reversing this process—of forcing the

evolved cell populations (e.g., T_6) back into normal patterns of growth—seems quite small. Both individuality and probable irreversibility characterize the tumor at this stage. At the same time, the phenomenon of genetic instability persists, thus permitting further variance. When patients are treated in attempts to destroy the malignancy, the neoplastic cells' capacity for further mutation allows them to develop resistance to treatment, and replaces the sensitive population that was killed by therapy. This is a rather discouraging prospect for therapeutic programs directed at tumor eradication.

Having introduced the model and some of its implications, we will now consider in more detail some of the key steps in tumor development.

INITIATION OF NEOPLASIA

This first step in tumor development, initiation, currently is the focus of intensive research. Because it is difficult to decipher underlying initial steps through the study of fully developed malignancies, much of this work is conducted in tissue culture. Cells are treated in vitro with viruses or chemicals to "transform" them into cells with malignant characteristics. In some cases, the transformed cells are transplanted into animals to test their tumorigenicity.

Several agents are capable of transforming cells in vivo or in vitro. Both experimental studies in animals and epidemiologic studies in man indicate the existence of a variety of carcinogenic substances. Various kinds of radiation, both ionizing radiation (e.g., x-rays, gamma rays, neutrons) and ultraviolet rays from the sun, are carcinogenic. A variety of chemicals also have this capacity. We are exposed to some of them occupationally; others are inhaled, as by cigarette smoking. Viruses also can induce cancer, at least in animals and it seems probable that this is also the case for some human tumors. Individual inherited genetic factors may facilitate the effects of one or more of these carcinogens in some people. Tumors are not necessarily or exclusively initiated by one particular agent; the first step in neoplasia may result from the interplay of several factors.

There are at least three fundamental questions about the initiation of cancer for which answers are uncertain. First, the primary event acts like a mutation, a heritable change induced by an alteration in the genetic material of the cell. It seems increasingly likely that all carcinogenic factors act through a common pathway by producing a change in the DNA of the cell. Nevertheless, the exact nature of that change is unknown. In fact, it may vary in different tumors. The alteration may range from gross structural rearrangements in the genetic material (e.g., gains, losses, or rearrangements of whole chromosomes or segments of chromosomes) to point mutations of a single gene. It may even involve, at the earliest stage, changes in regulatory genes that are potentially reversible and that do not involve an actual structural change in the genetic material.

A second problem is that the critical gene product or products in neoplastic transformation have not yet been discovered. Assuming that mutation has occurred in a cell that becomes neoplastic, the key structural or metabolic change in the cell that results from that mutation has yet to be identified. Thus, the precise molecular alteration that confers upon the cell the ability to respond abnormally to growth regulatory mechanisms is unknown, and it may vary in different tumors.

Much evidence seems to indicate that the critical gene product may often involve one or more molecules at the surface of the cell. These may be receptors involved in normal growth regulation. To regulate growth, an external signal must impinge on the cell. That signal, in some way, is passed from the surface of the cell through the cytoplasm to the nucleus, and it ultimately instructs the DNA to divide or not to divide. Many observations made on transformed cells in tissue culture point to changes in glycoprotein molecules on the surface, and portions of these glycoproteins may be receptors for local growth regulation.

For years, a uniquely absent or uniquely present molecule in the cancer cell has been sought. It seems increasingly probable, however, that early differences between neoplastic and normal cells are quantitative, not qualitative. For instance, surface receptors on a transformed cell simply may be modified in their number or arrangement so that the cell fails to respond adequately to regulatory signals. Such cells, then, have an enhanced probability for continued growth as compared to normal cells. The term "unrestrained growth" is commonly but imprecisely applied to neoplasia. Tumor cells are restrained, particularly in the early stages of their evolution. They still respond to normal growth regulation to some degree. But even a small abnormality in cellular responsiveness to growth regulation may be adequate to allow the population to begin to expand as a tumor.

A third major unknown concerns the mechanism of local growth regulation. For example, how do epithelial cells grow back to cover an injury and then stop without overgrowing? In contrast to the relative absence of information about local growth regulation, a fair amount is known about distant control. For example, hormones that circulate in the blood and stimulate or regulate growth at distant sites by binding to cell surface or cytoplasmic receptors have been well characterized. The means by which these hormonally-induced signals are transmitted to the nucleus to instruct cells to divide or not to divide is understood in some instances. Data on *local* growth control, however, is fragmentary. There is some evidence on stimulatory factors, such as epithelial and nerve growth factors, and also limited information on factors that specifically inhibit cell division when adequate numbers of mature cells are present. These inhibitory factors, or chalones, are substances that probably are produced by mature cells and act to terminate division in immature cells of the same type. As a corollary, a decrease in chalones would permit further cell division. The inference, then, is that cell division may result not only from stimulation but also from the absence of inhibition.

Such locally active substances are difficult to study. Because they must act over a short time and distance, they are highly labile and rapidly inactivated. Were they to function otherwise, chaos would result as they travelled throughout the body stimulating or inhibiting growth. The vast amount of new information generated in the last few decades includes substantiation of the intricate complexity of mammalian cells and tissues. Interacting networks operating at the level of the individual cell as well as between cells create a formidable labyrinth. The normal factors that determine growth and differentiation remain poorly understood. Without additional insights into these physiologic mechanisms, it is difficult to determine how a cancer cell, particularly early in its development, can be altered slightly and then go on to grow abnormally.

An important fact to bear in mind with regard to the initial step in neoplasia is that the triggering mechanism may be considerably separated in time from the ultimate proliferation of tumor cells. When a carcinogenic agent produces a genetic change or mutation in a potentially neoplastic cell, the effect will not become apparent until the cell divides. Bone marrow cells and the epithelium of the gastrointestinal tract are constantly proliferating to replace aged normal cells. Alteration in these cells is registered fairly promptly. Conversely, liver and kidney cells divide only rarely, and may not divide at all unless injury or some other stimulus triggers the division. A long latent period tends to occur before the effects of mutation become apparent. That may be one of several reasons for the characteristic latent period between exposure to a carcinogen and the appearance of a tumor in an individual. Other factors certainly play a role, but whatever the basis, latency is a major problem for epidemiologic studies. It is difficult to determine specific causes of human cancer when the carcinogenic exposure may have occurred 20 or more years earlier.

Some mouse experiments provide an interesting example. If a mouse is irradiated under certain conditions, no tumors will develop in the liver. If half of the liver in a normal mouse is removed surgically, the remaining liver cells will start to divide and eventually will regenerate the missing tissue. Once the liver grows back to normal size, the cells cease dividing. Local growth factors operate to turn off these cells, and no liver tumors result. However, if the mouse is irradiated, and the liver then partially resected, even two years later, regeneration will be followed by the development of liver tumors. Thus, until some sort of nonspecific promoting event transpires to cause the cells to divide, the effects of carcinogenic mutations induced earlier by radiation will not become manifest.

PROGRESSION OF NEOPLASIA

The previous discussion has addressed the earliest stage of tumor development. As defined in the model (Fig. 1–1), a population of cells with a selective growth advantage begins to expand locally. Whether this population of cells becomes malignant depends on the acquisition of additional properties at subsequent steps of evolution following T_1. Most important is the ability to invade and to metastasize, the classic definition of malignancy. Cancer cells have the capacity to separate from their brethren and to invade adjacent normal tissue, including thin-walled vessels, veins, and lymphatics. Single cells or clumps of cells travel to other sites in the body, forming satellite tumors (metastases).

The molecular basis of tissue invasion and metastatic dissemination is not fully understood. Changes that have been demonstrated in cancer cells include alterations in intercellular junctions, perhaps allowing malignant cells to separate more easily from one another than do normal cells. There are also data to suggest that cancer cells have diminished capacity to bind calcium to their surfaces. This results from changes in cell-surface molecules and may also be important in decreased intercellular adherence. Some malignant cells also show an increase in certain enzymes that digest one or more kinds of proteins, including collagen fibers. Through the production of collagenases, tumor cells may more easily move through tissue and vascular walls.

Another enzyme, hyaluronidase, may be a significant product of some tumors, breaking down elements in the supporting ground substance and thus allowing the malignant cells to invade more easily. Yet another tumor product is Tumor Angiogenesis Factor (TAF). Malignant cells appear to produce this substance in greater amounts than normal cells or benign tumors. It is postulated that through increased production of TAF, blood vessels proliferate into and around malignant tumors so that as they invade, adequate blood supply is generated. If a tumor is to continue to expand, an adequate blood supply is needed in order to deliver nutrients and oxygen. In fact, many rapidly growing tumors can outstrip their blood supply, and this results in necrosis of the entire center of the tumor.

Invasion of blood vessels and dislodgement of cells into the circulation is not enough to ensure the development of metastases. Circulating cancer cells must survive in the circulation and must lodge in a particular location that provides an appropriate environment. Platelets appear to be involved in this process. When tumor cells in circulation arrive at a particular foreign site, they may aggregate platelets around them, establishing a miniature clot in and around the tumor embolus. This clot seems to help to establish the tumor cells and to provide a fibrin meshwork upon which these cells can grow. Other, as yet undefined, characteristics of tumor cells, including surface antigens, are probably also important in metastasis formation.

In addition to invasion and metastasis, other characteristics are often associated with malignancy and tumor progression. Over time, cancers tend to grow with increasing rapidity. This is usually not because cells in the population go through the cell reproductive cycle more quickly than do normal cells. Rather, it represents an increase in the proportion of cells in the tumor that are dividing, and a decline in the percentage of cells that are "resting" or differentiating. The increased growth rate appears to result from a diminished response to normal growth regulation, in that fewer and fewer cells within the population react to signals that would normally instruct them to stop dividing and to differentiate—that is, to acquire the characteristics of a mature cell. Instead they remain in cycle and continue to divide and to increase the abnormal cell population.

Thus, as one might anticipate, the increased growth rate that occurs with tumor progression is associated with malignant cells that tend to look and act less and less differentiated. That is, progressively fewer cells in the tumor enter the maturation pathway to synthesize the specific products that characterize mature cells. Increasing numbers of cells remain in cycle, actively dividing and behaving like undifferentiated cells. In some tumors, this loss of differentiation may result from a mutation that actually "blocks" differentiation and leaves the cell no option other than to continue dividing. It remains uncertain how often an apparent block in differentiation is a primary event, or is secondary to the lack of response to normal inhibitory signals that control division.

Disturbances in cellular differentiation commonly lead to bizarre phenomena in cancer cells. Certain tumors begin to produce substances that normally are expected only from other tissues. For example, some squamous cell lung cancers synthesize a blood-calcium–elevating hormone that is similar to parathormone, resulting in significant clinical problems. Some tumors alter their surface glycoproteins to the point that the body recognizes them as foreign antigens and mounts an immunologic response to the cells, albeit usually an ineffective one. Thus far, it has not been possible to capitalize upon this immune recognition of cancer cells and to manipulate host defenses successfully in efforts to destroy the malignancy.

Abnormalities in cellular metabolic pathways are another feature of the progressively altered genetic makeup of tumor cells. In general, cancer cells tend to lose those pathways that are related to making specialized products of differentiated cells, and show a variable increase in the activity of pathways related to cell division. Unfortunately, as our model would predict, these alterations tend to vary in each tumor, and uniform patterns have not been found. The hope remains to discover a key biochemical change in cancer cells that sets them apart from normal cells. With this knowledge, it should be feasible, at least in principle, to design a chemotherapeutic regimen that would exploit this difference and kill cancer cells while sparing normal cells.

The problem persists, however, that if there is a critical bio-chemical change early in the evolution of malignancy, it will be obscured over time in a host of subsequent alterations. To sort these out and to isolate the clear signal from the background noise is indeed difficult. Those seemingly consistent patterns of bio-chemical abnormalities that have been reported generally have proved illusory on closer examination. For instance, many far-advanced tumors show increased anaerobic glycolysis. In the 1920s and 1930s, this was thought to be the hallmark of cancer. Later research showed that it probably simply reflected selection, in rapidly growing tumors, of a neoplastic population most capable of surviving in the environment of reduced oxygen resulting from inadequate blood supply. Modern technology now permits sophis-ticated assessment of subtle changes in the biochemistry of early cancer, but thus far no exploitable consistent alteration has been found.

Much of the evidence that tumor progression results from sequential genetic alterations in cancer cells is based on chromo-some studies of tumors. New karyotypic changes have been ob-served to appear over time, associated with changes in tumor prop-erties, but this relationship is variable in different tumors and in different patients.

Another aspect of tumor progression concerns the phenome-non of heterogeneity. The word "clone" implies that most tumors arise from a single cell. This might suggest that all of the cells in a tumor are the same at any given time, that the population is homogeneous. This is not the case. Heterogeneity, not homogene-ity, characterizes virtually every cellular property that has been investigated in advanced tumors. Our model (Fig. 1–1), and the supporting chromosome data, provide one explanation. Although one population of cells may predominate, there persists within the tumor residual subpopulations from earlier stages of its develop-ment. Moreover, as the process continues, the potential for vari-ance increases. Therefore, it is not surprising to find heterogeneity even in a clonal population, as defined. Unfortunately, this het-erogeneity complicates attempts to identify specific metabolic, an-tigenic, or other properties of the cell that might be exploited for treatment.

CLINICAL IMPLICATIONS OF CLONAL EVOLUTION

The model of cancer evolution described above affords some insights into attempts to control, treat, and cure metastatic dis-

.ease. The control of cancer is most effectively accomplished today by prevention, through identification of environmental elements that contribute to triggering the initial transformation of normal cells to cancer cells. Reduction in the number of chimney sweeps virtually eliminated scrotal cancer two centuries ago. The carcinogenic hazards of the aniline dye industry have been reduced, and a subsequent decline in related bladder cancers has occurred. Asbestos exposure, which is responsible for some cases of lung cancer and mesothelioma, is under continuing attack as a health hazard. Efforts are being made to eliminate heavy exposure to chemicals and radiation that have been documented in epidemiologic and experimental studies as important contributing factors in several human cancers.

Cancer prevention, however, is not simply a matter of scientific identification of carcinogens. Prevention intrinsically is a social, cultural, political, and economic issue. Consider, for example, the social, political, and economic ramifications of attempts to control the two best-documented causes of cancer in humans: cigarettes (lung cancer) and sunlight (skin cancer). Control of these causes requires major personal and cultural changes in lifestyle. The social and economic implications for the tobacco and recreation industries and for numerous satellite industries such as advertising and cosmetics are profound. Similar considerations apply to many occupational exposures to carcinogens.

Preventive measures that can be accomplished with greater facility and with less personal and social sacrifice are unfortunately often measures that would control relatively few tumors. Saccharine may be a good example of a possibly carcinogenic agent that has received attention disproportionate to its tumorigenic potential. Even had saccharine been banned, the reduction in the incidence of bladder cancer probably would have been minimal (and difficult to identify).

Although some carcinogens have been identified and are controllable, at least theoretically, the long latent period characteristic of tumor evolution makes it difficult to recognize and eliminate from the environment all or even most carcinogenic agents. The problem is complicated by inherited genes which may influence the susceptibility of particular individuals to specific agents. Nevertheless, progress may occur as subpopulations at increased risk are identified and counselled, leading to changes in behavioral patterns.

In view of our limited ability to prevent all cancers, early diagnosis and eradication must remain an important goal. Localized tumors can be removed surgically. If, however, the cancer has invaded widely or metastasized, other means are required. Radiation therapy, chemotherapy, or a combination of the two are employed to destroy cancer cells by irreversibly damaging their genetic material. The limitation here is that interventions that alter DNA in tumor cells also kill normal cells. Further, some cancer cells remain in the body following radiation or chemotherapy. What is required is therapy with selective capacity—therapy that can differentiate between tumor and normal cells and destroy only the former.

Despite ongoing testing of thousands of chemicals, despite increasing sophistication in biochemical investigation, and despite an expanded variety of tumors available for study in recent years, therapy capable of this differential effect has not been found. In view of what is known about the biologic, biochemical, and genetic characteristics of cancer cells, as discussed in the context of our model, it seems unlikely that an agent exists with the capacity to identify and kill only tumor cells and all tumor cells. Even if a specific difference was identified for a particular type of cancer, thereby allowing the development and application of therapy for that specific tumor, that cellular difference and that selective therapy might well not pertain to other neoplasms. The hope for a single agent, effective against a wide spectrum of cancers, is as unlikely to be fulfilled as was the hope for a single antibiotic useful against all microorganisms.

Immunologic attack remains a promising alternative approach, although research in this area to date has been disappointing. Evidence has accumulated to indicate that most tumors do generate some kind of immune response from the host. To a limited degree, the host attempts to eliminate a tumor much in the way that it attempts to eliminate a foreign kidney or skin graft.

Immune attack may be the specific means to rid the body of the remaining malignant cells that cannot be removed surgically or destroyed chemically or with radiation without killing the patient. Unfortunately, analogous to the situation in the cancer cell itself, the immune system is infinitely more complicated than it initially appeared to be. It is a highly complex, interlocking network of cells and cell products that feed back on one another in both inhibitory and facilitating ways. The present state of knowledge is such that attempts to stimulate the immune system in a patient with cancer may do more to interfere with the patient's existing immune response against the tumor than to improve it.

Much more knowledge of the workings of the immune system is required before it can be manipulated confidently to the benefit of patients.

Finally, one other therapeutic possibility which is appealing should be mentioned. It is based on the concept that neoplastic transformation in some cases may be partially or totally reversible. Rather than attempt to eliminate all existing cancer cells, the hope would be to manipulate the tumor environment in order to force the tumor cell population back into a normal balance between growth and differentiation. Experiments conducted under special circumstances have shown that malignant cells can be induced into normal patterns of growth and differentiation. For example, malignant mouse tumor cells were implanted into early, four-cell mouse embryos. In some of the mice that grew to adulthood, some normal tissues were found to have been derived from the tumor cells. Thus, in this setting, the tumor cells did function normally. Similar studies conducted with chemical and viral agents also suggest the potential reversibility of some neoplastic cells to normal cells.

Because cancer cells usually do retain the genetic information contained in their normal predecessor cells (although often scrambled), it is at least theoretically possible that cancer cells could be forced back into normal patterns of behavior. For most of the common cancers, however, this seems unlikely considering their long process of selection through multiple steps and mutations before becoming clinically evident. To be effective, reversibility would have to occur in virtually every cancer cell. If but a single malignant cell remained unchanged, it might well, through its continuing growth advantage over normal cells, reconstitute the tumor. As more is learned about local growth regulation, this approach may be useful in certain kinds of neoplasms. It may prove useful, for example, in those leukemias that seem to have few acquired genetic alterations. For most of the common cancers, however, the chances of success by this route appear small.

Thus, some fundamental questions about normal growth and differentiation remain, confounding our efforts to understand the process of cancer and to manipulate that process to the patient's benefit. The selective growth advantage of the tumor cell, its capacity to metastasize, and its genetic lability, in addition to the fact that available therapies do not differentiate between normal cells and cancer cells, all make it difficult to cure most of the common malignancies that are not surgically resectable. The end product of these factors in many cases is progressive evolution of tumors to clinically terminal stages of disease.

SUGGESTED READINGS

1. Cairns, J.: Cancer: Science and Society. San Francisco, W.H. Freeman, 1978.
2. Pierce, G.B., Shikes, R. and Fink L.: Cancer: A Problem in Developmental Biology. Englewood Cliffs, New Jersey, Prentice-Hall, 1978.
3. Pitot, H.: Fundamentals of Oncology. 2nd Ed. New York, Marcel Dekker, 1981.
4. Nowell, P.: The clonal evolution of tumor cell populations. Science, *194*:23, 1976.

Chapter 2

Common Medical
Complications

Peter A. Cassileth

Terminal malignant disease, by definition, is disease that has progressed beyond the point at which care aimed at remission or tumor regression is feasible. This condition may exist for days, weeks, or months. The period of survival in a terminal state is highly variable, eluding prediction and ready statistics. The patient's precise clinical status within the spectrum of advancing disease should determine the scope and direction of clinical intervention. However, professional bias often competes with such objective clinical determinants of care. Impending death is foreign to our goals, framework, and training; a tendency to withdraw from the case or to sustain futile aggressive efforts frequently supersedes the more rational, but professionally painful, focus on the patient's clinical status and needs. Palliative care is neither the absence of care nor the provision of passive care. It is active intervention of a specific, goal-oriented kind.

A great deal can be done to counteract or ameliorate the clinical problems of terminal disease. Appropriate interventions here, as during other stages of illness, require investigation, management, and professional involvement. Continuing action and participation not only contribute to the quality of the patient's remaining life; they also signify the physician's willingness to remain with the patient when fears of abandonment exacerbate the patient's physical and mental distress. The reluctance of many clinicians to fulfill this aspect of their role explains in part the growth of hospice in this country.

DIAGNOSTIC STUDIES

An initial problem in terminal care concerns the need for investigative studies on which to base treatment decisions. A critical question is whether the results of a study will potentially alter the patient's management. In clinical practice generally, efforts are made to determine the etiology of symptoms before treatment is initiated; however, tests and procedures required to document symptom etiology in terminal patients may cause more discomfort than is warranted by the information to be gained. Drawing a blood sample should cause minimal and tolerable discomfort, for example, but the benefit of barium enema evaluation in a debilitated patient may not merit the intrusion and discomfort induced by the procedure itself. In diagnostic evaluation, then, a balance must be struck between the importance of particular diagnostic data and the physical, emotional, and financial cost of obtaining them. Whether the patient is days, as opposed to months, from death becomes an important factor in such decisions.

Although clinical problems in terminal disease may derive directly from the malignancy, such problems frequently are due to indirect causes such as residual effects of previous surgery, chemotherapy, or radiation therapy. Further, patients in advanced stages of malignant disease may be receiving numerous medications, and the interactions between the different drugs that result from this polypharmacy can produce additional symptoms and problems. The clinician who adopts a nihilistic stance, holding that there is little or nothing to be done for the terminal patient, may attribute all problems to spread of the disease itself and may permit simple and readily manageable symptoms to go untreated. Many symptoms are amenable to correction with minimal evaluation and relatively non-discomforting means.

It is a striking feature of terminal illness that problems can be caused by one or many factors. It is a challenge to the physician's skill and a test of commitment to unravel the contributory features and to proceed appropriately. Some of the general problems faced by patients with advanced malignancies are discussed below. Specific treatment approaches are given in Chapter 17, and some of the most common problems are detailed in chapters devoted to their review.

WASTING

Wasting and malnutrition typically accompany advanced malignant disease. Despite the common misperception, wasting is not caused by the cancer's eating away body parts. Similarly, the fact that a growing cancer competes with organs and tissues for nutrients is rarely a significant factor in malnutrition. Occasionally, through the rapid turnover of cells, tumors may accelerate the body's metabolic demands to the point that nutrients and calories are consumed more rapidly than they are ingested. Uncontrolled diabetes mellitus, exacerbated by stress or corticosteroid administration, can also cause weight loss. In the majority of cases, however, weight loss and wasting are due to dysfunction of the gastrointestinal tract and to appetite changes. Decreased food intake and/or impaired capacity to absorb and utilize food result. Varying degrees of nausea with or without vomiting is another major cause of decreased food intake and subsequent wasting. A wide range of factors can contribute to nausea, including narcotics administered for pain.

APPETITE

Anxiety and/or depression due to disease progression and its prognostic implications can destroy appetite. However, other focal physical problems also play an important role. Tumor that originates in or spreads to the gastrointestinal tract can directly alter gastrointestinal physiology with resultant anorexia. Infiltration of the stomach or pancreas is also associated with the symptom of early satiety. Cancer of the pancreas also causes a specific aversion to protein foods, especially red meat. Metastases to the liver or hepatic disease of diverse causes leads to a spectrum of changes, from loss of appetite to nausea and vomiting. Similarly, even partial obstruction of a portion of the gastrointestinal tract from external tumor compression can initiate reflex changes that lead to diminished desire for food.

Poorly managed pain in and of itself can cause virtually total loss of appetite. Under these circumstances, the size of the tumor mass does not directly correlate with the extent of wasting; relatively small deposits of tumor in a bone may cause severe pain that can result in major weight loss over a relatively short period of time.

Metabolic dysfunction induced by liver or renal damage because of organ infiltration, obstruction, or drug-induced injury can play a major role in inanition. Uremia, acidosis, and accumulation of "middle" size molecules, of as yet uncertain nature, in renal failure make the patient ill. Impaired hepatic glycogenolysis and gluconeogenesis as well as reduced glycogen stores oblige reliance on protein and fat catabolism for energy. Decreased aerobic glycolysis leads to anaerobic metabolism of glucose with lactate accumulation. All of these changes contribute to systemic acidosis, anorexia, and nausea. Central nervous system dysfunction due to these metabolic derangements, to brain metastases, or to the toxic effects of fever and cardiopulmonary difficulties, diminish or eliminate the desire for food.

The importance of improving appetite and enabling the patient to eat as normally as possible cannot be overestimated (see Chapter 11). The loss of the ability to eat and to enjoy food is a major detriment to the patient, and to observe wasting is devastating both to the patient and the family. Patients are better able to cope with small amounts of food; often a full plate appears overwhelming and this can further diminish whatever appetite remains. Patients should be offered foods according to their personal preferences. Despite the bias that bland foods are better tolerated in this setting, patients are more likely to accept spicy or rich foods. Anorexia and nausea often can be alleviated with moderate doses of cortisone, prednisone, or other glucocorticoids. The mechanism of action of the glucocorticoids is unclear, but probably involves effects upon areas of the central nervous system responsible for appetite control at hypothalamic and cortical levels. Mood elevation and increased appetite usually result.

FEVER

Poor nutrition can result from fever, which is caused most often by infection, but also can result from the tumor itself. Hodgkin's disease, non-Hodgkin's lymphoma, and several solid tumors, such as disseminated breast or pancreatic cancer metastatic to the liver, can induce fever. Aside from causing anorexia, the hypermetabolic state increases calorie consumption and accelerates weight loss. Tumor-induced fever is largely prostaglandin-mediated. Thus, aspirin, corticosteroids, or the non-steroidal anti-inflammatory agents such as ibuprofen (see chapter 17), which are potent prostaglandin synthesis antagonists, can be of value. All of these agents have side effects. Aspirin and the non-steroidal anti-inflammatory agents impair platelet function and cause gastric irritation with increased risk of hemorrhage. Nevertheless, in numerous patients, their regular use eliminates fever totally, a result which is of such dramatic value to the patient that the potential hazard is warranted.

SWALLOWING PROBLEMS

Many patients suffer from a dry mouth syndrome due to decreased saliva production. The presence of saliva bears importantly on taste; food must be partly dissolved in order to be recognized by taste buds. Inadequate saliva, therefore, impedes the perception of taste and interferes with normal food intake. Changes in the mouth and in taste sensation also lead to markedly diminished enthusiasm for eating; it is uncomfortable even to think of eating when the mouth is severely dry and one is unable to taste food.

Radiation therapy to the area of the oropharynx and several chemotherapeutic agents damage the oral mucosa, atrophy the salivary glands and cause mucositis. Protracted periods of mouth breathing may contribute to these problems. These patients also suffer from changes in gums and teeth, and are prone to develop dental caries and gingivitis. Infections in the gum and pulp follow, contributing further to mouth discomfort and predisposing the patient to systemic infection. Granulocytes, along with the mucosal lining cells, are necessary to protect against local invasion by the teeming anaerobic bacterial flora of the mouth. Neutropenia from chemotherapy or marrow invasion by tumor thus facilitates ulceration of the mouth. Prednisone, with or without existing neutropenia, leads frequently to painful candidal mouth ulcers. Nystatin (Mycostatin) lozenges or mouthwash is useful in this setting.

A painful mouth thus can become an added deterrent to maintaining nutrition. Simple and direct means of counteracting this problem include wetting the mouth with ice chips and applying a lubricant or salve. Topical anesthetics, such as lidocaine (Viscous Xylocaine) or diphenhydramine (Benadryl) solutions, can be used to alleviate pain. They are not satisfactory, however, because they substitute for a painful mouth one that has no sensation at all. The relief obtained is brief and the absence of sensation does little to improve appetite.

Esophagitis from radiation injury, candida infection, or acid reflux causes pain on swallowing. Swallowing Viscous Xylocaine provides relief. Monilial esophagitis is not cured by nystatin orally and requires daily parenteral low dose (10 to 15 mg) amphotericin B intravenously. To the degree that acid regurgitation plays a role in esophageal pain, cimetidine (Tagamet) and antacids provide significant benefit.

DEFICIENT FOOD ABSORPTION AND METABOLISM

Nutrition may be deficient even in the face of adequate ingestion. Small intestine injury from radiation enteritis or diminished small intestine surface area secondary to surgical excision impairs nutrient absorption. Impairment of the pancreatic secretion of bicarbonate, which neutralizes stomach acid secretions, prevents establishment of optimal pH for small intestinal enzyme activity. The absence of pancreatic lipase precludes the formation of the micelles necessary for the absorption of fats and fat soluble vitamins. The result is steatorrhea; administration of oral pancreatic enzyme supplements corrects this problem. Fat malabsorption due to obstruction of biliary flow, either extra- or intra-hepatic, is less easily managed. A diet rich in medium-chain triglycerides, rather than long-chain fatty acid triglycerides, circumvents this problem. Liver dysfunction arising from drug toxicity or metastases may so impair hepatic intermediary metabolism that inadequate utilization of fats, amino acids, and carbohydrates results.

Diarrhea results from malabsorption, whether induced by radiation enteritis or steatorrhea. In the latter case, the failure of bile salt absorption causes bile acid irritation of the small intestine. Antibiotics that alter the normal bowel flora can cause diarrhea as well. Carcinoid tumors (and, rarely, pancreatic cancers) secrete biogenic amines which can stimulate intestinal peristalsis. The net result of diarrhea is rapid intestinal transit time and decreased opportunity for nutrient absorption. Cramps and abdominal bloating accompany the diarrhea and in the debilitated patient create the hazard of incontinence. Most patients and families can manage the progressive wasting of terminal disease and the constricted range of activities, but the indignity of fecal incontinence is difficult to handle. The use of antispasmodics such as diphenoxylate (Lomotil) and/or codeine (or stronger narcotics) reduces the symptoms of diarrhea. In the incontinent patient, timed administration of small enemas (Fleet's) allows scheduled evacuation of the lower rectosigmoid and decreases the risk of random unannounced emptying.

CONSTIPATION

A peculiar facet of constipation is that it often appears as diarrhea and/or incontinence. Attempts to treat these manifestations only compound the problem. Fecal impactions, which result from progressively dehydrated stools becoming hard and large and obstructing the flow of stool, can cause these symptoms. The more liquid portions of the stool above the mass ooze around it and cause incontinence which is interpreted as diarrhea. A simple rectal examination discloses the presence of hard stool. Treatment consists of fracturing the mass by digital manipulation followed by enemas.

Constipation is infinitely more common among patients with advanced cancer than diarrhea, and the presence of apparent diarrhea should alert the clinician to constipation as the probable cause. Generally, such patients are minimally active, which tends to slow down intestinal contractions; and usually the small amount of food ingested is low in bulk, which diminishes peristaltic reflexes. Many patients are on narcotics, even the least potent of which markedly inhibit intestinal motility. For a person in good health, constipation may be a relatively minor nuisance. For patients in advanced stages of disease, however, many small problems contribute to major misery. Management of constipation is easily accomplished.

Prevention is preferable to correction, however, and constipation should be treated prophylactically as an integral aspect of routine management for patients at risk, including all patients on narcotic analgesics. Stool softeners, laxatives, and bulk formers help to maintain normal bowel function. Improvement in this area also is associated with improvement in appetite.

MANAGEMENT OF CACHEXIA

Chapters 11 and 17 discuss specific means of treating the wasting syndrome in cancer patients. Some interventions against malnutrition and wasting are not appropriately applied in terminal disease. A nasogastric tube, for example, is unacceptable and unnecessary for most patients. Insertion of a nasogastric tube, despite its small size, becomes a major treatment decision in advanced malignant disease. If the problem is not absorption or obstruction, such patients essentially can be force-fed despite lack of appetite. One must question, however, whether this is desirable given the constellation of that patient's needs and the quality of existence.

Similar considerations apply to the problem of inadequate fluid intake. Dehydration can be corrected by intravenous fluid administration, but this is usually unnecessary. The effects of dehydration are perceived by patients symptomatically as thirst. Moistening of the mouth with ice chips, as noted previously, is a simple and effective approach. Dehydration proceeds inexorably to hypovolemia and renal failure. Among the mechanisms of death in the cancer patient, uremia is associated with relatively little distress for the patient who gradually slips quietly into coma. Electing not to treat dehydration can be an acceptable option in some circumstances.

PAIN

Pain, as is true of other symptoms in advanced malignancy, has multiple potential etiologies. It is not entirely academic to consider the mechanism of pain production, because it may dictate a means of specific relief. Any hollow organ of the body, such as the intestine, the bile ducts, or the ureter, may be obstructed with tumor, creating back pressure and swelling behind the area of obstruction. This triggers severe pain because pain sensors in hollow viscera respond to distention. Compromise of the lumens of these organs by the primary tumor or its metastases causes major difficulties because of organ dysfunction and pain.

Tumors that infiltrate sensory nerves cause extraordinary discomfort as can tumors that infiltrate serosal surfaces, such as the parietal pleura or peritoneum. Bone pain from primary bone cancer or bony metastases comes from the expansile pressure of the tumor not on the bone itself, but on the bone lining. Sensory nerves that supply the endosteum and periosteum respond to stretch. It is not erosion of bone, but rather distortion of the lining membranes, that causes pain. For example, a patient with kidney cancer was in a moderate amount of pain because of a large tumor deposit in the scapula. He then noted one day that the pain in his shoulder was entirely gone. The tumor finally had erupted from the bone and now was easily palpable as a subcutaneous mass; the decompression had relieved the pain. Although the patient perceived this as a measure of improvement, it was in fact a measure of advancing disease. Of course, bone pain or distorted bone architecture can lead secondarily to spasm of periosseous musculature in a reflex response to hold the painful parts immobile. Muscle spasm over the damaged parts may then become a major component of the patient's pain which can respond to heat and muscle relaxants.

Like bone, brain tissue is not sensitive to pain. Pain associated with cranial and intracranial cancer emanates from sensory nerves in the scalp, the lining of the calvarium, and the meninges. In brain tumors or metastases to the brain, a certain amount of edema almost invariably develops, enhancing expansion and swelling caused by tumor deposits. Meningeal distention causes pain. At the same time, cerebrospinal fluid flow may be obstructed by tumor, causing increased pressure (internal hydrocephalus) because fluid production continues in the face of limited capacity for reabsorption. In massive pharmacologic doses, corticosteroids such as prednisone or cortisone can markedly reduce the swelling that occurs around these tumor deposits. This provides substantial pain relief and even reversal of neurologic deficits.

Corticosteroids in high or moderate doses over periods of time have a number of side effects that are virtually irrelevant in patients with terminal malignancy since such patients will not receive the drugs for long enough periods of time for the side effects to be expressed. Thus, fat deposition, increased facial hair in women, acne, diabetes, cataracts, stomach ulcers, and osteoporosis are not important side effects to consider. Except in patients with a history of ulcers or preexisting diabetes, glucocorticoid side effects do not represent significant contraindications to glucocorticoid administration in patients with terminal disease.

The degree of pain experienced by the patient is modulated by the patient's pain threshold. A particular pain stimulus is perceived as extreme by some patients, but as only moderate by others. Patients with advanced cancer are under severe psychologic stress, and stress lowers pain thresholds, so that relatively modest degrees of pain may be perceived as severe.

Patients' lifestyles are severely constricted, given a general lack of distractions, decreased opportunities for personal or business interactions, and few obligations to meet or plans to make. With little to occupy their thoughts other than continuing concerns about the cancer, their pain often is magnified. The distractions of day-to-day life in the healthy individual often deter pain perception until the evening, when one relaxes and prepares for sleep. Progressive isolation—physical isolation caused by inability to perform job tasks or work in the home, interpersonal isolation caused as the people interacting with the patient find communication increasingly difficult, and sensory deprivation caused by growing loss of input from outside—exacerbates the perception of pain. Therefore, approaches to pain relief must occur simultaneously on several levels.

Pain is a meaningful symptom to patients in that they tend to regard it as a sign of worsening disease. Even cancer patients who are not terminal and whose pain can be readily managed may equate the presence of pain with proximity to death. There is also an associated sense of helplessness, a perception that pain is a weakness, which is magnified in patients accustomed to independence and self-control. Such patients may experience severe pain but do not complain of it, because acknowledging the extent of pain and the need for exogenous relief is unacceptable to them. In this regard, it is helpful to provide patients with some insight into the origins of pain. It is not enough, nor is it necessarily true, to explain only that pain is due to the cancer. It is much more helpful to determine the exact reason for the pain and to tell the patient what is generating it. With this information, patients can come to grips with the problem and regain some sense of control.

At the same time, patients should be provided with a conceptual framework that permits them to accept narcotics without emotional distress. One useful approach, particularly for patients concerned about narcotic addiction, is to provide analogies to other symptoms and their treatment. For example, one can explain that aspirin taken for headache or fever prior to illness, or medications taken to control the cancer or to deal with other symptoms, were perceived correctly as useful and appropriate therapies for medical problems. Explaining that pain should be viewed as another symptom requiring medication and that narcotics can be safely discontinued when the cause is otherwise eliminated should assist patients to gain perspective on pain management.

Many patients also believe that once pain begins, it will worsen inevitably and progressively, and that it cannot be handled. The anxiety over what the pain means, which can be relieved by explaining its source and implications, plus the anxiety over whether the pain can be controlled at all, increases the perception of pain. Reassurance is a helpful and important adjunct to therapy. Then, of course, relief must be provided. Etiology and management are considered below (see also Chapter 17).

Although the patient may not be a candidate for aggressive treatment, interventions relieve specific problems with minimal discomfort to the patient. A painful area of bone, for example, may be treated with a small amount of radiation therapy in a short course to shrink the tumor, relieve the pressure, and diminish the pain. This obviously need not be the same dose of radiation therapy applied to eradicate cancer from that site.

On occasion, a surgical maneuver to relieve a specific symptom may be appropriate. For example, extra-hepatic biliary obstruction by tumor can cause painful biliary colic and pruritus, and create the potential for progressive liver failure and ascending cholangitis. It may be amenable to surgical correction by a shunting procedure or T-tube placement. In appropriately selected patients, postoperative pain and morbidity is acceptable in return for relief of symptoms and the opportunity for substantial time free of these symptoms and problems.

In recent years, minimally hazardous, nonsurgical means of alleviating pain have been developed. Two examples are the passage of a catheter through common duct obstructions by percutaneous transhepatic biliary cannulation; and the use of intra-arterial emboli to infarct hemorrhagic or painfully enlarging masses in renal cancer.

The goal of pain management is not alleviation, but elimination of pain. This goal can be accomplished through the administration of medication around the clock. If obliged to wait until the pain recurs, the patient begins to experience a little pain, and decides not to complain. Then the pain becomes somewhat more intense, and finally the pain becomes severe and medication is requested. Now, starting from this heightened level of pain and anxiety, the patient must wait for the medication to be swallowed, digested, and absorbed. During this time, pain escalates and only later does some pain relief occur. This is not optimal pain management. It is preferable to determine a dose that renders the patient pain-free on a regular-dosage basis. This approach eliminates the anticipation of pain, and also enables the patient to maintain a sense of control.

Striking a balance between adequate pain relief and undisturbed mental function poses a problem in some patients. Particularly in some older patients, narcotic analgesics may produce unacceptable sedation or drowsiness. In treating patients in their 70s and 80s, one should try a scaled-down dosage first. Older people metabolize drugs differently than do younger patients. Their response to drugs is not readily predictable, and cerebrovascular arteriosclerosis and modestly impaired brain function may leave them with little reserve. It is preferable to try a minimum dose first and to escalate it later, rather than to attempt a full dose initially and find the patient comatose or disoriented with a toxic psychosis. Some patients prefer to have tolerable pain rather than experience the confusion or disorientation that may accompany total pain relief. This is an individual matter that requires resolution in terms of the particular patient. The goal is to find a level of analgesia that will not produce unacceptable degrees of sedation, confusion, or disorientation. In only a few patients does agonizing pain require constant narcosis (e.g., by continuous I.V. morphine infusion).

INFECTION

Patients with cancer rarely die of the direct effects of cancer, in other words, of tumor invasion of a vital organ. Most patients with cancer die because wasting and inanition lead to decreased host resistance, and patients succumb to bacterial infection. Endogenous infection, from the patients' own normal intestinal flora, usually is responsible for the development of pneumonia or urinary tract infection with or without bacteremia. Bacterial egress from normal sites into the blood is facilitated by neutropenia, altered mucosal surfaces induced by therapy or tumor invasion, and mechanical alterations from obstruction or surgery. Because of the cancer patient's diminished capacity to mobilize an inflammatory response, the symptoms of infection are often limited to fever and rigors and focal findings are reduced.

One must consider how aggressively to seek out and treat the source of infection. Evaluation requires urinalysis, chest roent-

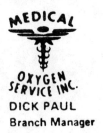

MEDICAL

OXYGEN
SERVICE INC.
DICK PAUL
Branch Manager

1230 Hemingway Drive
South Commercial Park
Ft. Myers, Florida 33907
1-813-489-1877
Toll Free 1-800-282-5579

NOV 5
4.00

Dentist

Complete Line of Durable Medical Equipment

genogram and cultures of blood and urine, and therapy involves antibiotics pending results of the studies. Whether these investigations and treatment are warranted depends on the patient's overall status. In patients whose quality of life is severely diminished, the physician may decide not to treat the infection or, as an intermediate step, to eschew the studies and to provide oral antibiotics only.

In the hematologic malignancies, in contrast to solid tumors, infection is more likely to occur earlier in the course of advanced disease and is more frequently related to neutropenia. Here, treatment of infection may allow additional months in reasonable comfort. Therefore, infection usually is treated in patients with advanced hematologic malignancies, but often introduces a critical decision point for patients in advanced stages of other malignant diseases.

DYSPNEA

Impaired oxygen transport is a common problem in patients with advanced cancer. Hypoxemia obliges the patient to work harder physically through the increased activity of respiratory muscles. The effort is fatiguing and disabling. When difficulty in breathing is severe and compensatory cardiopulmonary mechanisms inadequate, the patient experiences a terrifying sensation of suffocation.

The causes of dyspnea are manifold. Efficient transfer of oxygen and carbon dioxide at the pulmonary alveoli is accomplished across the single layer of lining cells to the juxtaposed alveolar capillaries in the interstitium of the lung. This delicate interstitial meshwork is a common site of metastases for all cancers. The spread of cancer through and along pulmonary blood vessels (whether the malignancy initiated in or spread to the lung from another primary site) ramifies throughout the lung fields in an interstitial pattern seen on chest roentgenogram and inaccurately called lymphangitic spread.

Increasing the distance between the alveolus and capillary reduces oxygen transport and leads to increasingly labored, fast, and deep breathing to effect improved gas exchange. Thickening of the interstitium can occur because of tumor deposits and/or because of neoplasm-induced desmoplasia and local edema, reducing lung compliance. Enhanced respiratory effort is then required not only because of the hypoxemia, but also because of the work required to expand relatively inflexible lung tissue.

Similar stiffening of the mechanics of respiration can occur when tumor infiltrates the lining of the chest. Mechanical stiffening of the chest wall decreases mobility and contributes to breathlessness. The nodules of primary tumor or metastases seen on roentgenogram may be few and small, yet patients may have a great deal of trouble breathing. The chest roentgenogram visualizes only gross tumor deposits and underrepresents the widespread microscopic (but functionally important) spread of tumor throughout the lungs. Marked impairment of the mechanics of breathing, therefore, may not correlate with what appears on roentgenogram.

Tumor deposits in the pleura further impair pulmonary function. The inflammatory response to serosal infiltration causes pleuritic chest pain. The automatic response is splinting of the chest wall, which limits motion and respiration. The serosal cells of the pleura secrete small amounts of fluid. Tumor infiltration increases fluid formation and, depending on its location, also may block reabsorption. Pleural fluid accumulates, compressing lung tissue and enhancing respiratory decompensation.

Factors not directly related to the cancer may also contribute. A patient with lung cancer and a long history of heavy smoking, for example, commonly has some degree of underlying chronic obstructive pulmonary disease. Even relatively minimal tumor deposits can significantly decrease lung function when superimposed upon impaired function caused by chronic bronchitis and/or emphysema. Underlying problems may be so severe that further compromise by a relatively small burden of pulmonary cancer or bronchial obstruction causes decompensation. In addition, patients with cancer and arteriosclerotic cardiovascular disease may lack adequate cardiac reserve in response to hypoxemia with the development of superimposed congestive heart failure and pulmonary edema.

Anemia may be present—caused by the disease, bleeding, or myelosuppression from therapy—and it can contribute to impairment of compensation for respiratory insufficiency. The body's adaptive responses to anemia are so substantial that most patients do not require transfusions for hemoglobins of 8 g/dl or more. However, patients with lung dysfunction may have so much distress that transfusion is necessary at these levels. Transfusion with packed red blood cells increases oxygen-carrying capacity and decreases the work of breathing. Nasal oxygen, supplied by bedside tanks or small portable tanks worn on the shoulder, is often a most effective means of relieving dyspnea, especially when combined with small doses of morphine to relieve anxiety.

It is usually impossible to reduce the extent of pulmonary parenchymal tumor invasion in terminal cancer patients. However, ancillary approaches such as correction of congestive heart failure, red blood cell transfusions for anemia, and supplemental oxygen delivery are useful. Pleurisy caused by thoracic wall invasion can be alleviated by analgesics to improve respiratory excursion. If dyspnea results in part from bronchial obstruction, radiation therapy to a relatively small area of involvement may open the occluded airway.

Pleural effusions, on the other hand, can be approached directly. Several factors should be considered before therapy is initiated. Diagnostic thoracentesis with a small gauge needle should be performed to look for malignant cells. If the patient is not in congestive heart failure and the fluid is a transudate without cancer cells, then the accumulation is due to lymphatic obstruction. In this circumstance, the patient may benefit from radiation therapy to the central mediastinum or hilar nodes. If the fluid is chylous, the explanation usually is entrapment of the thoracic duct in the posterior mediastinum where the duct crosses from right to left at the level of the T5 vertebral body. Even without a demonstrable mass on chest roentgenogram, blind irradiation of this area can relieve chylothorax.

In most cases, pleural fluid is serosanguineous and cancer cells are present. Thoracentesis provides immediate relief of lung compression and should ease dyspnea. However, in many patients parenchymal lung invasion is so substantial that the pleural effusion, in fact, is a relatively minor component of dyspnea. Thoracentesis in these patients, even of substantial volumes of fluid, yields surprisingly little benefit. If the patient improves, the problem of how rapidly fluid will reaccumulate remains. The physician and patient may be faced with the prospect of repeated thoracenteses.

Whether such maneuvers are worthwhile in an individual patient depends on projections of life span and on concomitant clinical problems. Decisions should be based on the potential for substantial relief from thoracentesis. A tap may leave the patient comfortable for weeks or months, or fluid could reaccumulate the next day.

Although thoracentesis is not terribly painful, it is uncomfortable physically and conceptually. Moreover, regardless of the rate of fluid production, there is a tendency for fluid to flow back into the chest following a tap, thereby drawing fluid from the intravascular volume and causing hemodynamic alterations that add to the patient's discomfort.

If repeated taps are required, sealing the pleural surface by the intrapleural instillation of sclerosing agents, such as nitrogen mustard or tetracycline, should be considered. This technique is effective in 60 to 65% of patients but has some significant drawbacks. For maximum effectiveness, an intrapleural chest tube must be inserted and connected to suction in order to drain the chest of fluid and to bring the pleural surfaces closely together. The chest tube remains in place for 5 to 7 days, generally causing discomfort, and intrapleural therapy elicits an inflammatory response with pleurisy and fever which takes up to a week to subside. Moreover, if the procedure fails, the patient is left with loculated pleural effusion that is no longer amenable to relief by thoracentesis. As with other interventive measures in the terminally ill patient, all ramifications of the patient's general disease status and survival outlook must be taken into account.

High doses of narcotics, especially morphine, decrease dyspnea and reduce the patient's sense of suffocation. Levels of narcotics adequate to achieve this aim depress the body's respiratory drive. Patients with poor oxygen delivery then breathe less well at a time when they can ill afford it, and hypoxemia worsens. Nevertheless, because dyspnea is such a terrifying symptom, high doses of narcotics may be warranted in advanced stages of disease when survival expectation is brief.

HEMATOLOGIC COMPLICATIONS

Mild degrees of anemia are common in advanced cancer. In most patients, hemoglobins stabilize in the range of 8 to 10 g/dl. At this level, cardiorespiratory compensation usually is adequate to keep the patient asymptomatic at ordinary levels of physical activity. Transfusions thus are rarely necessary except in the case of cardiac and/or pulmonary dysfunction. In the solid tumors, despite extensive disease (including marrow infiltration), significantly impaired myelopoiesis is rare. Most, if not all, terminal care can be handled in the home and on an outpatient basis.

In contrast, varying degrees of pancytopenia occur frequently in patients with advanced hematologic neoplasms. The need for red cell transfusions for severe anemia, platelet transfusions for thrombocytopenic bleeding, and therapy for sepsis due to neutropenia plagues patients' final days, making consistent outpatient management difficult. For these patients the extensive requirements for supportive medical care make a dignified death, free of encumbrances of medical technology, a rare occurrence.

BLADDER DYSFUNCTION AND INCONTINENCE

Incontinence of urine (or of stool, as discussed earlier) is exceedingly difficult for the patient and family to handle. Urinary incontinence may be caused by neurologic damage through tumor invasion of the sacral autonomic plexus or by compression of the spinal cord. The bladder may contract too frequently, resulting in spontaneous urination before the patient is aware of the need to urinate. The bladder may empty poorly, creating substantial pelvic pressure and causing the bladder periodically to empty small amounts of urine (overflow incontinence). Inadequate emptying may be caused by underlying prostatism or by obstruction of the urethra due to pelvic deposits of tumor, especially in patients with cancer of the cervix or prostate.

Incontinence may be exacerbated in the elderly or debilitated patient whose level of awareness and perception is impaired. Tumor deposits in and around the bladder or urethra can cause irritation and frequent emptying. Rapid relief by a drainage procedure is required when obstruction is severe or total.

All of these circumstances of dysfunction predispose the patient to bladder and kidney infection. For symptomatic patients, urinary cultures and sensitivities guide selection of antibiotics which can be given orally. For patients found to have asymptomatic bacteriuria, no treatment is required. In patients with frequent symptomatic urinary tract infections, mechanical problems should be corrected, if feasible. Where it is impossible to repair urinary tract drainage mechanics, long-term administration of a trimethoprim-sulfamethoxazole (Bactrim or Septra) combination suppresses urinary tract bacteria for long periods of time. This technique is useful in preventing repeated septic episodes in the terminal patient.

Depending on the exact cause of incontinence, various interventions may be attempted. If the problem stems from poor bladder contraction and inadequate emptying, medication such as bethanechol (Urecholine), which facilitates bladder contraction, may help to achieve complete emptying. Mechanical rather than physiologic treatment is applied for structural abnormalities or if medical therapy fails. For random emptying of the bladder, an external condom sheath to catheter drainage is useful in men, but is often troublesome because of the penile irritation that occurs. An indwelling urethral catheter with a closed drainage system is frequently required. The catheter is uncomfortable initially, but sensory adaptations soon extinguish perception of its presence. It is certainly preferable to the disagreeable manifestations of incontinence.

EXTRACELLULAR FLUID RETENTION

The accumulation of extracellular fluid is another common event in advanced malignant disease. Precisely where fluid localizes in the body is determined in part by gravity. Fluid tends to accumulate in the lower portion of the body and legs in patients who spend most of their time sitting up, and to collect along the back in supine patients. Causes relate to lymphatic or venous obstruction; hypoproteinemia; liver, renal, or cardiac failure; and the administration of corticosteroids or other medications that cause salt and water retention such as indomethacin (Indocin) and estrogens.

Patients with advanced malignancy and wasting synthesize proteins poorly because of inadequate food intake and diminished hepatic function. The oncotic pressure of protein helps to retain water in the circulation, so that hypoproteinemia, whatever its cause, worsens fluid retention. Diuretics are of use but may have limited effect because of hypovolemia and reduced glomerular filtration rate. Intravenous albumin infusion briefly (until it is metabolized) raises intravascular oncotic pressure but its effects are so transitory that it has little value. The only durable means of improvement is to enhance nutritional status, which may or may not be feasible or appropriate in the individual patient.

Lymphatic or venous obstruction usually leads to fluid accumulation distal to the obstruction. Lymphatic blockade almost invariably is due to tumor masses impeding the flow. If localized, radiation therapy may help, otherwise little can be done except to elevate the edematous part. In both lymphatic and venous obstruction, diuretics offer little and mobilization of accumulated fluid usually requires doses that will induce unacceptable levels of hypovolemia. Although the genesis of venous obstruction may be tumor compression, its major effects are due to venous thrombosis. If tumor mass reduction is not possible, the thrombosed vein will not recanalize.

The liver's reserve capacity is so vast that significant compromise of function by tumor invasion occurs only with massive replacement of liver by cancer. When this occurs, death follows shortly. If liver failure appears to play a role in fluid retention, it is usually due to hepatic or portal vein thrombosis rather than to neoplastic liver infiltration. Diuretics and anti-aldosterone agents can be beneficial. Prolonged common duct obstruction can lead to biliary cirrhosis, but in most patients common duct obstruction can be relieved surgically or by cannulation (see above).

Peritoneal tumor implants can cause ascites. All of the considerations regarding therapy of pleural effusions apply here. The side effects of ascites include degrees of intestinal hypoactivity approaching ileus, painful abdominal distention, and respiration-impairing elevation of the diaphragm. Diuretics are rarely of value in this setting. Peritoneal taps and/or intraperitoneal chemotherapy may be employed. For patients with one or more months of projected survival, placement of a Leveen shunt is a useful maneuver. The surgically established subcutaneous catheter drains ascitic fluid from the abdomen into the atrium. As long as it remains patent, it alleviates the distressing effects of massive ascites.

Renal failure is another cause of fluid retention. If it is due to intrarenal causes, little correction can be expected. On the other hand, supervening metabolic factors such as hyponatremia, hyperuricemia, hypercalcemia, or urinary tract infection can be managed with marked improvement in renal function. If lower urinary tract obstruction cannot be mechanically relieved from below, establishing a catheter in the renal pelvis through a nephrostomy can reverse renal shutdown, allowing months of useful life. The usual indication for this procedure occurs in women with squamous cell carcinoma of the cervix. Cervical cancer tends to infiltrate pelvic structures extensively, invading urethra and bladder early in the disease, whereas distant metastatic disease is a late phenomenon. Nephrostomy placement in these patients saves them from a premature death in renal failure.

HYPERCALCEMIA

Hypercalcemia causes important but easily correctable metabolic dysfunction. In addition to multiple bony metastases, a common cause of hypercalcemia is a hormonal substance, similar to parathormone, produced by some tumors. Tumors, primarily lymphoid neoplasms, also release prostaglandins or osteoclast activating factor which causes bone resorption and hypercalcemia. Calcium deposition in bones is a dynamic process that is aided by weight bearing and muscle action. In the absence of these stimuli, bedridden patients tend to lose bone calcium. This demineralization enhances the tendency to hypercalcemia.

Hypercalcemia results in constipation, nausea, vomiting, renal dysfunction, and mental changes ranging from confusion to coma and seizures. If hypercalcemia is not considered, these symptoms are readily and incorrectly attributed to other problems, such as nausea and vomiting from liver metastases or medication, confusion from brain metastases, renal dysfunction from obstruction, or constipation from narcotics. The importance of investigating cause before attempting treatment is particularly evident here.

Rapid partial correction is achieved by hydration orally or intravenously with saline. Once hydration is achieved, calciuresis can be forced with intravenous furosemide (not with thiazides because they cause calcium retention). However, stimulating excessive urination in debilitated patients or in patients with renal or urinary dysfunction is not an optimal solution. Further, intravenous volume loading is contraindicated in elderly terminally ill patients with anemia, and/or borderline cardiopulmonary function because of the risks of precipitating congestive heart failure. A better approach is the use of the chemotherapeutic drug, mithramycin. Minute doses intravenously inhibit osteoclast activation, virtually without side effects. Serum calcium levels fall to normal levels within 24 to 48 hours, and doses can be repeated two or three times a week, if necessary.

Moderate dose corticosteroids can reduce hypercalcemia in some tumors, particularly breast cancer and myeloma. Mobilizing the patient from bed to chair or from chair to ambulation is a helpful maneuver if feasible. If pain prevents mobility, analgesics should be administered to allow increased activity.

DEATH FROM LIVER OR KIDNEY FAILURE

Death from liver failure is not uncommon in malignant gastrointestinal disease. The metabolic effects induced by liver failure lead to changes in sensorium causing drowsiness, stupor, coma, and death through a gentle and slow progression. It is a relatively asymptomatic means of dying. The same is true of kidney failure, wherein uremia induces a similar sequence of central nervous system events.

As the sensory level falls, the patient may not perceive what is happening, but a variety of noncognitive and reflex activities, such as groans and odd movements, may occur. Families tend to attribute significance to these random motions and utterances. They may infer, for example, that the patient is calling them, or is in pain or otherwise distressed. This is rarely the case in the presence of severe central nervous system dysfunction.

Central nervous system depression evolves systematically, with loss of the higher cortical centers preceding loss of the more primitive medullary centers that control respiration, heart rate, and blood pressure. Thus, well before fatal dysfunction supervenes in these essential control mechanisms, the higher intellectual centers cease to operate. The physician should explain to family members that the observed behaviors are random events without meaning. The loss of relatedness to the family that accompanies this kind of death is balanced by the opportunity for a relatively peaceful and painless death.

Note, however, that the level of suppression or depression in central nervous system function can be misjudged. One should not assume that the patient is totally oblivious; even when patients seem immobilized and unaware, it is possible that they still may hear and understand what is said around them. It is better to behave as if the patient were capable of cognition than to risk depersonalizing and distressing a still-aware patient. It is always wise, no matter what the patient's apparent mental status, to continue to communicate and to assume that the patient's level of perception permits comprehension.

FINAL DECISIONS

The decisions of when and how to intervene in the problems of the terminal patient require thoughtful analysis of multiple aspects of the patient's existence and disease status. It is well to anticipate expected supervening problems and to discuss them with the patient and family so that some of the responses to complications may be determined before hand. For example, a difficult decision is faced when the patient is symptomatic from a urinary tract infection, pyelonephritis, pneumonia or bacteremia, all of which are associated with high fever and will cause death if left untreated or inadequately treated. The question then is when to treat and when to withhold intervention. Oral medications frequently will not suffice and therapy involves diagnostic study, placement of intravenous lines, and administration of antibiotics for many days in the hospital.

Whether or not this is appropriate represents a critical decision. What is the quality of daily life? To what status will the patient be returned if the infection is corrected, and for how long? The standard of care for management of terminally ill cancer patients must involve this layer of considerations lest the discomfort of the care itself become an added burden for the dying patient. At the same time, the multiplicity of factors potentially giving rise to symptomatology must be carefully assessed to avoid attributing all that occurs to irremediable cancer, thus missing the opportunity to improve the quality of the patient's last days.

SUGGESTED READINGS

1. Abeloff, M.D. (ed.): Complications of Cancer: Diagnosis and Management. Baltimore, Johns Hopkins University Press, 1979.
2. Anderson, C.B., Philpott, G.W., and Ferguson, T.B.: The treatment of malignant pleural effusions. Cancer, 33:916–22, 1974.
3. Bayly, T.C., et al.: Tetracycline and quinacrine in the control of malignant pleural effusions: a randomized trial. Cancer, 41:1188-92, 1978.
4. Benson, R.C. et al.: Radioimmunoassay of parathyroid hormone in hypercalcemic patients with malignant disease. Am. J. Med., 56:821–26, 1974.
5. Black, L.F.: The pleural space and pleural fluid. Mayo Clin. Proc., 47:493–506, 1972.
6. Blackman, M.R., Rosen, S.W., and Weintraub, B.D.: Ectopic hormones. Adv. Intern. Med., 23:85–113, 1978.
7. Cartwright, G.E.: The anemia of chronic disorders. Br. J. Haematol., 21:147–52, 1971.
8. Costa, G.: Cachexia, the metabolic component of neoplastic diseases. Cancer Res., 37:2372–75, 1977.
9. DeWys, W.D.: Anorexia in cancer patients. Cancer Res., 37:2354–58, 1977.
10. DeWys, W.D., and Walters, K.: Abnormalities of taste sensation in cancer patients. Cancer, 36:1888–96, 1975.
11. Dilworth, J.A., and Mandell, G.L.: Infections in patients with cancer. Semin. Oncol., 2:349–360, 1975.
12. Donaldson, S.S.: Nutritional consequences of radiotherapy. Cancer Res., 37:2407–13, 1977.
13. Garnick, M.B., and Mayer, R.J.: Acute renal failure associated with neoplastic disease and its treatment. Semin. Oncol., 5:155–65, 1978.
14. Gilbert, H.A., et al.: Evaluation of radiation therapy for bone metastases: pain relief and quality of life. Am. J. Roentgenol., 129:1095–96, 1977.

15. Greenberger, N.J., and Shellman, T.G.: Medium-chain triglycerides: physiologic considerations and clinical implications. N. Engl. J. Med., *280*:1045–58, 1969.
16. Gybels J., Adriaensen, H., and Cosyns, P.: Treatment of pain in patients with advanced cancer. Eur. J. Cancer, *12*:341–51, 1976.
17. Hendrickson, F.R., and Sheinkop, M.B.: Management of osseous metastases. Semin. Oncol., *2*:399–403, 1975.
18. Kechel, S.J., and Rodriquez, V.: Acute infections in cancer patients. Semin. Oncol., *5*:167–80, 1978.
19. Lazor, M.Z. and Rosenberg, L.E.: Mechanism of adrenal steroid reversal of hypercalcemia in multiple myeloma. N. Engl. J. Med., *270*:749–55, 1964.
20. Levine, A.S., Graw, R.G., and Young, R.C.: Management of infections in patients with leukemia and lymphoma: current concepts and experimental approaches. Semin. Hematol., *9*:141–155, 1972.
21. Light, R.W., Erozan, Y.S., and Ball, W.C.: Cells in pleural fluid: their value in differential diagnosis. Arch. Intern. Med., *132*:854–60, 1973.
22. Mazzaferri, E.L., O'Dorisio, T.M., and LoBuglio, A.F.: Treatment of hypercalcemia associated with malignancy. Semin. Oncol., *5*:141–54, 1978.
23. Mundy, G.R., et al.: Evidence for the secretion of an osteoclast-stimulating factor in myeloma. N. Engl. J. Med., *291*:1041–46, 1974.
24. Myers, W.P.L.: Differential diagnosis of hypercalcemia and cancer. CA *27*:258–72, 1977.
25. Perlia, C.P., et al.: Mithramycin treatment of hypercalcemia. Cancer, *25*:389–94, 1970.
26. Posner, J.B.: Diagnosis and treatment of metastases to the brain. Clin. Bull., *4*:47–57, 1974.
27. Rodriguez, V., Burgess, E.M., and Bodey, G.P.: Management of fever of unknown origin in patients with neoplasms and neutropenia. Cancer, *32*:1007–12, 1973.
28. Saunders, C.M., Ed.: The Management of Terminal Disease. Chicago, Year Book Medical Publishers, 1978.
29. Schein, P.S., et al.: Nutritional complications of cancer and its treatment. Semin. Oncol., *2*:337–48, 1975.
30. Seyberth, H.W., et al.: Prostaglandins as mediators of hypercalcemia associated with certain types of cancer. N. Engl. J. Med., 293:1278–83, 1975.
31. Sickles, E.A., Greene, W.H., and Wiernik, P.H.: Clinical presentation of infection in granulocytopenic patients. Arch. Intern. Med., *135*:715–19, 1975.
32. Theologides, A.: Nutritional management of the patient with advanced cancer. Postgrad. Med. J., *61*:97–101, 1977.
33. Wilson, F.A., and Dietschy, J.N.: Differential diagnostic approach to problems of malabsorption. Gastroenterology, *61*:911–31, 1971.
34. Zucker, S., Friedman, S., and Lysik, R.M.: Bone marrow erythropoiesis in the anemia of infection, inflammation and malignancy. J. Clin. Invest., *53*:1132–38, 1974.

Chapter 3

Central Nervous System Manifestations

Donald H. Silberberg

Nervous system complications resulting from advanced cancer or its treatment often limit the patient's quality of life. Continued survival with severe impairment of neurologic function is the least desirable of outcomes. Because over one third of patients with malignancies develop neurologic manifestations or complications, and because pain is a problem for many more, the recognition and management of brain, spinal cord, nerve, and muscle dysfunction are crucial. Increasingly successful therapy makes it possible to correct neurologic impairment in many terminal cancer patients. Neuro-oncology is receiving increasing attention from neurologists; however, the number and pressing nature of the problems involved demand the attention of all physicians who treat patients with malignant disease.

For the purposes of discussion, the neurologic manifestations and complications of cancer are divided into those that result directly from tumor invasion or metastatic growth, and those that arise at a distance from the cancer itself. Complications of treatment are then reviewed.

METASTASES

Most metastases of non-neurologic cancers to the nervous system travel by way of the arterial circulation. This fact dictates their distribution, which in general parallels the rate of blood flow to the various parts of the nervous system. The spread of prostate and other pelvic malignancies by way of the paravertebral venous plexus of Batson is an exception; invasion and spread through these veins lead primarily to a vertebral body and base of skull distribution for these particular tumors. A further distinction must be made between tumors that metastasize hematogenously to the parenchyma of the brain or spinal cord, and those that spread first to bone and extend secondarily to contiguous nervous system structures. Any of the manifestations described below may be early or late developments in the patient with cancer.

Intracranial Metastases

Approximately 15% of patients who die of cancer have brain metastases at autopsy.[1] More than half of these patients will have experienced neurologic symptoms during life.

Intraparenchymal Tumors

The most common tumors that metastasize to brain are pulmonary carcinomas, although tumors arising in virtually every other organ may do so. Not infrequently, a patient presents with intracranial metastasis as the first manifestation of a cancer arising outside of the nervous system (usually lung cancer). Almost 90% of brain metastases occur within the cerebral hemispheres, about 10% in the cerebellum, and less than 2 or 3% in the brain stem. In approximately half of patients, intracranial tumors are multiple when first discovered. The number of metastatic deposits varies with the primary site; thus, lung carcinomas commonly produce a single metastasis whereas metastases from melanomas almost always are multiple.

Most commonly, neurologic dysfunction referable to the site of metastasis is the first symptom of its presence. For example, a left parietal lobe tumor compromises speech and produces a right hemiparesis, hemisensory deficit, and often a right visual field deficit as it compresses the normal structures in that area. Symptoms and signs of increased intracranial pressure, which may accompany or precede focal neurologic dysfunction, include increasing generalized headache, nausea and vomiting, and episodic dimming of vision with increasing papilledema. The patient may develop persistent focal headaches prior to the development of increased intracranial pressure, caused by stretching of blood vessels, dura, or other pain-sensitive structures.

Fewer than 10% of such tumors announce themselves with the sudden appearance of neurologic symptoms. This can occur by the following mechanisms: 1) a tumor may trigger an epileptic seizure as its first manifestation; 2) as the metastasis enlarges and outgrows its newly developing intrinsic blood supply, it may undergo necrosis, leading to hemorrhage and rapid expansion of the tumor mass (most commonly in melanomas and bowel carcinomas); and 3) tumors occasionally occlude an intracerebral vessel, causing infarction of tissue distal to the site of occlusion.

Bear in mind that not all intracranial tumors that develop in patients with a known cancer diagnosis are metastases. Patients may develop benign intracranial tumors such as meningiomas and pituitary adenomas, quite independent of a primary malignancy elsewhere.

Diagnostic Studies

The indicated diagnostic studies are dictated largely by the degree of involvement of other organ systems. The patient who has at least several months of comfortable life ahead, based on the status of other organ systems, requires careful evaluation in order to design therapy. The increasing resolution of the computerized tomographic (CT) brain scan makes it the leading diagnostic laboratory method. Metastatic tumors are identified as spherical areas of increased or decreased density in relation to surrounding brain, usually surrounded by a zone of edema. Edema disrupts the blood-brain barrier, often yielding an area of ring-like enhancement on CT scan after intravenous injection of a contrast material. Alternatively, the entire tumor may enhance. Occasionally an arteriogram may be needed to distinguish a metastasis from a meningioma or other benign tumor.

At times, lumbar puncture is required to measure spinal fluid pressure, to obtain fluid for cytologic examination for malignant cells, or to exclude a concurrent infection. Because the CT scan can assess the possible risk of brain herniation, a CT scan should always be obtained when the possibility of increased intracranial pressure exists, before a lumbar puncture is considered. Herniation is unlikely if the ventricular system is not compromised.

Tumors Arising from Bone and Dura

Metastases arising from seeding of bones or meninges compress adjacent structures, producing local pain and/or local neurologic signs. For example, multiple cranial nerve palsies associated with visual field loss clearly indicate the presence of tumor at the base of the brain in the region of the sella turcica. Tumors over the convexity of the hemispheres often produce a seizure early in their course. Patients with metastases in this location often also have evidence of metastases to bone.

Treatment

Appropriate treatment may result in substantial improvement or even in cure of intracranial metastases. The decision of whether to treat and of what therapeutic goals to establish must be based on the status of the cancer and on its other manifestations in a particular patient. The most appropriate initial treatment for metastatic tumors usually is radiotherapy, to a total dose of 3000 or 3500 rad. Lymphomas and testicular cancers are among the most radiosensitive tumors. Relatively radioresistant tumors include melanoma and carcinoma of the bowel and kidney. Lung, breast, and ovarian cancers are intermediate in radiosensitivity. About 50% of the patients treated with radiotherapy regain normal neurologic function. Results are better for those with more radiosensitive tumors.

The CT scan provides an essential tool for determining the response to radiotherapy. This objective assessment should be used to complement clinical evaluation of the patient's progress.

It is often appropriate to use high-dose systemic corticosteroids to reduce the brain edema that surrounds metastatic tumors. Dosage adjustment is made subsequently, based on the patient's response and on serial CT scan studies. In many instances the use of corticosteroids is the most urgently needed of the various therapies available, because the reduction of edema occurs in hours, whereas radiation-induced shrinkage takes weeks. The prompt administration of corticosteroids thus can acutely reduce intracranial pressure and prevent herniation and compromise of vital brain stem functions. Corticosteroids are a powerful therapeutic tool and may be used successfully to preserve neurologic function for months despite continued tumor growth.

After commencing radiotherapy and corticosteroids, the patient is observed for tumor regression. In many instances, the tumor shrinks markedly and even disappears. Surgical removal may be considered for a solitary metastasis in an accessible area. Perhaps the most likely candidate for craniotomy is the patient with a solitary melanoma or bowel carcinoma metastasis in the right (non-dominant) cerebral hemisphere.

Many patients deteriorate neurologically despite CT evidence of complete disappearance or marked regression of their tumors. Such patients usually are suffering from metabolic encephalopathy from the systemic effects of malignancy. Under these circumstances, it is inappropriate to withhold treatment because of the belief that brain metastases have become uncontrollable (see following).

Spinal Metastasis

Spinal cord compression by cancer with consequent paraplegia and incontinence is usually the result of direct spread from a metastasis in a vertebral body. This complication occurs in about 5% of all patients with cancer.[2] Paraplegia or quadriplegia may progress slowly, even over months, or may progress to total paralysis within hours or days. In general, prognosis is better for those patients who have progressed slowly and worse for those who have developed total paralysis before treatment is instituted. Some form of treatment almost always is indicated because paraplegia and incontinence are deeply distressing to a conscious patient and require a major escalation in nursing care. For this reason, early recognition is essential, and each emerging symptom should be evaluated promptly.

Often the first symptom is back pain, sometimes starting as vague discomfort. Ataxia, leg weakness, urinary urgency or hesitancy, or more marked (radicular) pain may be the next symptom to develop. Symptoms are often worse with coughing or sneezing. The physician should perform a careful neurologic examination, obtain spine films of the appropriate regions, and proceed quickly to further x-ray studies if the symptoms persist or if abnormal neurologic signs are found. Traditionally, myelography has been the most effective means for locating epidural spinal cord compression and the rare instance of intraparenchymal spinal cord metastases. The increasing resolution of spinal cord, meningeal, and vertebral body structures that can be achieved with the newer generation of CT scanners adds a valuable imaging approach that supplements and may eventually replace myelography. We have found that the use of a water soluble radiopaque medium, such as metrizamide, provides useful combined myelogram-CT scan delineation of spinal cord tumors.

Treatment with high-dose systemic corticosteroids should be started *as soon as clinical suspicion* of spinal cord compression seems well founded. This should be instituted even before any radiologic studies are obtained. One need not be concerned that the radiologic findings will be obscured by therapy. Acute reduction of edema may preserve neurologic function, and the tumor will remain visible. Occasionally, intravenous mannitol is needed to induce a hyperosmolar state to provide rapid reduction in tumor-induced spinal cord edema.

The choice of treatment by radiotherapy, chemotherapy, or decompressive laminectomy depends on the patient's overall prognosis and the likelihood of a rapid response to a nonsurgical modality. Surgical treatment usually is reserved for those patients with relatively radioresistant tumors who have a block at a single level that is progressing. Such patients also should have adequate residual neurologic function and a life expectancy of more than two months.

Meningeal Spread (Carcinomatosis of the Meninges)

Not infrequently, carcinomas and lymphomas spread diffusely throughout the meningeal coverings of the brain and spinal cord. The usual manifestation of this complication is the dysfunction of one or more cranial nerves (or spinal nerves) with rather rapid progression to involve other adjacent nerve roots. The finding of even a single cranial nerve palsy in a cancer patient should always raise the suspicion of meningeal spread. Symptoms and signs often are bilateral and soon are accompanied by malaise, generalized headache, and sometimes other meningeal signs such as stiff neck and photophobia.[3]

The cerebrospinal fluid findings are useful in diagnosing meningeal carcinomatosis, but it is important to realize that similar findings may be produced by opportunistic infections such as cryptococcosis. Typically, cerebrospinal fluid pressure is normal or somewhat elevated. Total protein is elevated to levels of 80 to 150 mg/dl and the glucose is reduced to less than 45 mg/dl. Although spinal fluid glucose levels may be as low as 10 mg/dl one must realize that hypoglycorrhachia occurs in only half of patients with meningeal carcinomatosis. Obtaining a concomitant blood sugar is of little value. There is approximately a two hour lag between changes in blood and spinal fluid glucose levels. Moreover, the spinal fluid glucose will not fall below 45 to 50 mg/dl except in the face of severe and prolonged hypoglycemia. The spinal fluid cell count usually is increased in the range of 5 to 50 cells/mm³. Many of the cells will prove to be malignant on careful microscopic examination. On occasion, however, most of the cells will be lymphocytes secondarily generated by tumor-induced meningeal irritation.

Cytologic examination is valuable in distinguishing between meningeal carcinomatosis and chronic meningitis. Spinal fluid should always be sent for smears and cultures in search of bacterial and fungal organisms. A CT scan should be obtained in advance to rule out increased intracranial pressure that could cause uncal or brain stem herniation in response to the lumbar puncture. This hazard can be reduced by treatment with mannitol and/or corticosteroids just prior to lumbar puncture. The risk of losing large amounts of spinal fluid can be minimized by performing lumbar puncture with a small gauge needle.

Treatment with cranial and spinal radiotherapy and intrathecal methotrexate can be beneficial, producing clinical improvement that persists for the balance of the patient's life span.

Nerve Roots and Peripheral Nerves

Root or peripheral nerve entrapment may occur as an isolated neurologic complication. For example, local pelvic extension of cervical carcinoma often compresses part of the sacral plexus, leading to leg weakness and/or sensory loss. More commonly, the region of the brachial plexus is involved, either by tumor extension or metastasis or as the result of radiation neuropathy. Metastatic involvement of the brachial plexus typically produces severe shoulder pain radiating down the medial part of the arm to the elbow and sometimes into the hand. Weakness and sensory loss develop in the distribution of the cervical and upper thoracic nerve roots, producing sensory loss in fingers and weakness of the intrinsic hand muscles. Horner's syndrome with ipsilateral miosis and absence of facial sweating often occurs. The patient with chronic postirradiation changes in the brachial plexus experiences less discomfort, and Horner's syndrome is uncommon.

Pain

The pain that results from the distortion of local structures by cancer is, of course, mediated by the nervous system. To date, treatment methods have been relatively crude, reflecting our lack of understanding of pain physiology. Opiates and other analgesics are moderately effective, but often have side effects such as constipation and alteration of sensorium that must be managed (see Chapter 17). As our understanding of the biochemistry of endorphins, opiate receptors, and the pathophysiology of pain increases, many more specific pharmacologic agents will become available.

Neurosurgical procedures such as cordotomy are needed occasionally, to interrupt the pathways conducting pain.

NONMETASTATIC COMPLICATIONS

Central Nervous System and Meningeal Infections

Subacute and Chronic Meningitis

The altered immunologic status of patients with cancer (especially lymphoid cancers), sometimes leads to the development of meningeal infection with such opportunistic organisms as Listeria monocytogenes or Cryptococcus neoformans. Meningitis may be the first manifestation of the underlying malignancy, but it usually occurs in patients with established diagnoses. Because these are often indolent infections, symptoms are often present for days or weeks before a physician is consulted. Early symptoms include headache, malaise, and loss of appetite followed later by stiff neck, photophobia, and progressive loss of consciousness. The patient may describe night sweats and have a fever when first seen. Interference with cerebrospinal fluid circulation may lead to hydrocephalus as part of the clinical syndrome.

The use of the spinal fluid examination is discussed previously in this chapter in the section on meningeal carcinomatosis. Repeated lumbar punctures are usually required to establish the correct diagnosis and to monitor treatment. Treatment with amphotericin B, or with appropriate antibiotics, may eliminate the infection.

Brain Abscess

Infection by fungi such as aspergillus or mucor, or by parasites such as toxoplasma, may lead to localized collections of organisms and their products that mimic the symptoms and signs of metastatic tumors. They often may be distinguished from metastatic tumors by CT scan. The success in curing brain abscesses has increased enormously with the advent of CT scan monitoring and with more aggressive use of antibiotics.

Progressive Multifocal Leukoencephalopathy

The occurrence of multifocal brain and spinal cord white matter infection by a papovavirus is an uncommon complication that usually occurs in patients with metastatic cancer who have significant immunologic impairment.[4] This disorder produces hemiparesis, paraparesis, visual loss, or other focal signs that progress to death over the course of several weeks. This appears to result from alterations in immune responsiveness. The virus affects primarily the oligodendrocytes, the cells that synthesize and maintain myelin within the central nervous system. Spinal fluid examination usually is normal. The diagnosis may be suspected on the basis of the clinical presentation and confirmed by evidence of multifocal cerebral white matter lucencies on CT scan. No treatment is known.

Limbic Encephalitis

Encephalitis, limited to the brain stem and the deep midline structures including the limbic system, occurs as a rare complication of underlying malignancy.[5] This produces the rather rapid onset of brain stem dysfunction with loss of consciousness and is usually fatal. It is distinguished from progressive multifocal leukoencephalopathy because gray matter rather than white matter is involved. It is unusual for any of the known neurotropic viruses to produce encephalitis limited to the brain stem and other midline structures in adults who do not have an underlying malignancy.

Metabolic Encephalopathies

Patients with malignancy-produced hepatic or renal failure or other metabolic disturbances often develop dementia, hemiparesis, or alterations of consciousness. These symptoms and signs may be associated with difficulty in maintaining posture, which produces an irregular downward jerking of outstretched hands (asterixis). The electroencephalogram is a valuable monitor of cerebral dysfunction produced in this manner.

The recognition of metabolic encephalopathies in patients with cancer may be difficult, especially in those who also have intracranial metastatic tumors. In those patients, continuation or progression of neurologic dysfunction despite treatment of the metastases may lead the physician to assume that the treatment has failed. Often, careful assessment shows that tumor regression *has* occurred and that supervening problems such as uremia, hypercalcemia, or hyperosmolarity are responsible for increasing malaise and neurologic dysfunction. When a particular brain region has been previously injured by metastatic tumor, or a stroke, that region is more susceptible to dysfunction if a systemic metabolic disturbance occurs. Distinguishing between progressive tumor invasion of brain and metabolic encephalopathy is necessary for appropriate management.

Vascular Disorders

Patients with cancer may develop strokes as a complication of their malignancies or as a result of hypertensive or arteriosclerotic cerebrovascular disease. Occasionally, pulmonary metastases shed tumor emboli, producing occlusions of small cerebral vessels and infarction. Similarly, nonbacterial (marantic) thrombotic endocarditis often embolizes to intracranial vessels. Intracranial hemorrhages can occur as a consequence of thrombocytopenia or disseminated intravascular coagulation. Hyperviscosity syndromes can lead to arterial occlusions.

Remote Effects of Cancer (Paraneoplastic Syndromes)

Several rare nervous system manifestations of cancer are recognized; the pathophysiology of these disorders is unknown. These syndromes may be the first sign of the presence of a malignancy, but more commonly complicate the later course of a patient with cancer.

Peripheral Neuropathy

Clinical peripheral neuropathies develop in 2 to 5% of patients with cancer, most commonly with lung carcinoma (primarily small cell carcinoma), and less often with gastrointestinal malignancies and lymphomas. Electromyographic studies of patients with cancer have shown that subclinical neuropathy may occur in up to 50% of patients, so that this actually ranks as the most common nervous system manifestation of cancer.

The neuropathy may precede other evidence of the primary tumor by up to five or six years, although the usual interval is approximately six months. Less commonly, peripheral neuropathy develops after the diagnosis of carcinoma has been made. The onset usually is subacute with progression over several months, after which the symptoms may remain static. Rarely, symptoms start acutely. In some patients, the neuropathy can be severe and crippling. In several series the mean survival from onset of neuropathy to death was approximately 14 months.

The neuropathy is usually predominantly sensory with numbness and paresthesias of the extremities and often of the face. At times it is asymmetric in distribution. To the neurologist, facial neuropathy indicates the strong possibility of an underlying malignancy. Motor involvement with weakness and fasciculations occurs less commonly, and isolated motor neuropathies are rare. There is little tendency for improvement, even with successful treatment of the underlying malignancy.

Cerebrospinal fluid examination may be normal, but frequently shows elevation of spinal fluid total protein as high as 200 mg/dl. Electromyographic and peripheral nerve conduction studies are essential for accurate diagnosis.

A less common neuropathy of malignancy is an acute inflammatory polyneuropathy, producing the clinical picture of the Guillain-Barré syndrome. This has been reported particularly in Hodgkin's disease, and it does remit. A remitting and relapsing neuropathy has occurred in some patients with underlying malignancy.

Direct invasion of nerve roots and nerves by tumor cells may cause a symmetrical polyneuropathy in association with lymphoma and multiple myeloma, but is rare in association with carcinomas.

Dermatomyositis

Muscle weakness attributable to muscle inflammation and degeneration, associated with skin erythema (dermatomyositis) may be the initial manifestation of an occult malignancy when it presents in younger women and older men. This syndrome may complicate the course of any patient with an underlying malignancy. Muscle weakness usually progresses over several months and may lead to severe disability. It is usually more proximal than distal, at least initially, and occasionally appears in combination with peripheral neuropathy. This fact led to the erroneous concept of a "neuromyopathy," a term that still appears in some reviews. The most common underlying tumor is oat cell carcinoma of the lung in men and ovarian carcinoma or lymphoma in young patients. The disorder may improve with corticosteroid therapy, and instances of apparent remission have occurred after removal of a primary tumor.

Subacute Cerebellar Degeneration

Progressive ataxia of limbs and speech in a patient with malignancy may herald the uncommon occurrence of carcinomatous subacute cerebellar degeneration, usually in association with carcinoma of the lung. It causes progressive disability over the course of months to a year or two. The cause is unknown. Improvement following treatment of the primary tumor has been reported. Before concluding that this is the cause of progressive ataxia, one must exclude the much more common events of spinal cord compression by epidural metastases, tumor metastatic to the cerebellum, hydrocephalus caused by intracranial metastases, or sensory neuropathy.

Dementia

Although many cases have been reported, it is difficult to establish a clear association between the occurrence of dementia and an underlying neoplasm, because dementia on the basis of Alzheimer's disease or other unknown causes is a relatively common disorder. However, instances of presenile dementia, although not of the Alzheimer's type histologically, occur in association with malignancy, principally with carcinoma of the lung.

Acute Transverse Myelopathy

Rarely, subacute or acute necrosis of the spinal cord occurs in the absence of either direct metastases or infarction. This produces paralysis or paraplegia. No treatment is known.

Iatrogenic Complications

Chemotherapy

Peripheral neuropathy is a limiting factor in the use of some chemotherapeutic agents. It results from the effects of agents such as the vinca alkaloids on the neurotubules and other cytoskeletal elements in peripheral nerve. Sensory and motor dysfunction result. If it has not progressed too far, peripheral neuropathy improves when treatment by the offending agent is discontinued.

Progressive multifocal leukoencephalopathy (previously mentioned) is a rare occurrence in patients with cancer, but seems more likely to appear in those undergoing chemotherapy.

Another leukoencephalopathy occurs as a complication of treatment with methotrexate, usually in patients treated with intrathecal methotrexate over long periods of time. It also appears, however, in some patients receiving cranial irradiation combined with relatively brief courses of intrathecal methotrexate without prior brain radiation. The disorder may produce an aggressive myelopathy or an encephalopathy with bilateral signs and dementia.

Brain Irradiation

Radiation therapy to the brain may produce acute, subacute, or chronic side effects.[7] Acute symptoms occur during or immediately following a course of radiation therapy and are easily attributable to the therapy. These include the following: headache, meningeal signs such as photophobia, and stiff neck, fever, and worsening of neurologic signs. These side effects are transient. Subacute effects occur 6 to 8 weeks after radiation and include symptoms of headache, lethargy, and nausea and vomiting. These have been reported primarily in children with acute lymphocytic leukemia undergoing prophylactic brain irradiation and in adults treated for glioma. These symptoms can lead to the erroneous assumption that the patient has progressive CNS disease. Treatment with corticosteroids may hasten improvement, but the symptoms resolve spontaneously even if untreated. The distinction between radiation side effects and tumor progression can be made through analysis of serial CT scans.

Rarely, some patients who have received high-dose radiation to a treatment portal that includes the brain stem develop brain stem signs suggesting a demyelinating disorder. Chronic side effects of radiation therapy begin a year or more following therapy. Some patients develop necrosis of brain tissue which leads to a reappearance of signs originally attributable to the tumor. Asymptomatic cerebral atrophy is seen on CT scan in many patients who have had brain irradiation.

Spinal Cord Irradiation

Radiation myelopathy may be subacute or chronic. The subacute form begins 8 or 10 weeks after radiation therapy, usually to the neck, and is characterized by Lhermitte's sign, which is an electric shock-like sensation radiating down the back and into the arms and legs upon flexion of the neck. This may persist for several weeks and usually disappears. No treatment is needed.

Chronic radiation myelopathy occurs months to years after therapy. It may appear with the onset of a Brown-Séquard syndrome (ipsilateral limb weakness with contralateral loss of pain and temperature sensation). It may be painless or associated with radicular pain. A myelogram is necessary in such patients to rule out metastatic spinal cord compression. Unfortunately, radiation myelopathy may produce spinal cord enlargement, mimicking tumor, but can usually be distinguished from intradural metastatic tumor growth. Chronic radiation myelopathy is a progressive disorder. Treatment with corticosteroids may slow this progression.

Decisions regarding the treatment of patients with neurologic manifestations of cancer require an understanding of nervous system functions and careful consideration of the differential diagnosis of a given symptom or syndrome. The approach to treatment depends on residual and recoverable neurologic function and on the patient's overall status. The primary purposes of treatment are preservation of useful function and maintenance of comfort.

REFERENCES

1. Posner, J.B., and Chernik, N.L.: Intracranial metastases from systemic cancer. Adv. Neurol., *19*:575–587, 1978.
2. Posner, J.B.: Neurological complications of systemic cancer. *In* Symposium on Clinical Neurology: New Approaches to Old Problems. Med. Clin. North Am., *63*:783–800, 1979.
3. Little, J.R., Dale, A.J.D., and Okazaki, H.: Meningeal carcinomatosis, clinical manifestations. Arch. Neurol., *30*:138–143, 1974.
4. Weiner, L.P., et al.: Papovavirus of JC type and progressive multifocal leukoencephalopathy. Arch. Neurol., *29*:1–3, 1973.
5. Corsellis, J.A.N., Goldberg, G.J., and Norton, A.R.: "Limbic encephalitis" and its association with carcinoma. Brain, *91*:481–496, 1968.
6. Shy, J.M., and Silverstein, J.I.: A study of the effects upon the motor unit by remote malignancy. Brain, *88*:515–528, 1965.
7. Kramer, S., and Lee, K.F.: Complications of radiation therapy: the central nervous system. Semin. Roentgenol., *9*:75–83, 1974.

Chapter 4

Palliative Chemotherapy: Risk/Benefit Ratio

John H. Glick

The term "chemotherapy" is associated with cancer despite the fact that, strictly speaking, other therapy such as penicillin prescribed for a streptococcal sore throat is also chemotherapy. The word chemotherapy conjures up a variety of negative images: hair falling out, nausea, vomiting, and physical deterioration. Many patients and families perceive chemotherapy as a last desperate attempt to treat advanced cancer. Few equate chemotherapy with the opportunity to produce cure or disease regression in a patient with cancer. The extensive negative connotations of cancer chemotherapy are rooted in the personal or implied experiences of friends, in the lay literature, and in the early history of the development of anti-cancer drugs.

CHEMOTHERAPY: AN HISTORICAL PERSPECTIVE

Prior to 1945, many deaths occurred from tuberculosis and other infectious diseases. Sulfa drugs were available but were effective for only a limited number of bacterial infections. Toward the end of World War II, penicillin was marketed, and a host of effective antibiotics for all varieties of infectious diseases, including the once dreaded scourge of tuberculosis, followed rapidly. This kind of chemotherapy was the magic bullet that cured previously fatal illnesses. Further, antibiotic chemotherapy had few and rare unpleasant side effects.

At about this same time, the earliest antineoplastic agent appeared. This was nitrogen mustard, a drug synthesized as a by-product of efforts to develop chemical warfare weapons. The initial clinical application of nitrogen mustard occurred in a patient with lymphoma and yielded exciting results: the disease completely disappeared. Initial enthusiasm, however, was shortlived. The patient relapsed and was less responsive to the second attempt at treatment. In 1948, methotrexate was synthesized, enabling remissions in acute lymphocytic leukemia. Subsequently, 5-fluorouracil was developed, offering promise against colon cancer. Public expectations for a cancer cure were raised by initial reports of dramatic chemotherapy-induced remissions and heightened by the impressive progress against bacterial disease.

The new antineoplastic agents, however, failed to produce the cures hoped for. Furthermore, they frequently caused adverse reactions. Some negative side effects were intrinsic to the specific chemotherapeutic agents employed; others stemmed from the need for additional research to document optimal dosage levels and schedules. Not enough was known about the action and mechanism of these early agents to guide physicians in their use. Data were not then available to determine when in the disease process chemotherapy is best administered; how the drugs should be applied to maximum effect; and when to halt the regimen.

Unrealistically high public expectations quickly faded as patients with cancer were seen to become nauseated, bald, and emaciated while receiving chemotherapy and to die, confused or comatose, despite the treatment. Of these effects, only hair loss and transient nausea can be attributed directly to chemotherapy. Nevertheless, patients and families tended to blame the drugs rather than the tumor for what were actually the ravages of the disease itself. Thus, chemotherapy acquired a reputation for inducing rather than ameliorating illness. Occasionally, a new patient who is potentially curable with chemotherapy refuses treatment, saying, "My father died horribly from his treatment for lung cancer." In reality, what had been observed was a patient dying from lung cancer that had spread to the liver and caused nausea, vomiting, jaundice, malnutrition, and pain.

CHEMOTHERAPY: A CURRENT PERSPECTIVE

There are approximately 1,000,000 new cases of cancer in the United States each year. These include 300,000 cases of skin cancer and in situ cancer of the uterine cervix, which are 100% curable by surgical excision or local radiation therapy. This leaves 700,000 new cancer diagnoses annually. Approximately 70%, or 500,000, of these cancer patients present with localized disease, and approximately 56%, or 280,000, of these patients can be cured with surgery and/or radiation therapy. For three quarters of the 220,000 who are not cured by initial treatment and who are at high risk for recurrent cancer, chemotherapy potentially can prevent or delay relapse. Effective chemotherapy also exists for half of the 200,000 patients with metastatic disease at initial diagnosis.[1] Thus, prolongation of life and potential cure through chemotherapy are realistic goals for the management of many cancer patients at various stages of the disease process.

Research on cancer in animals provides useful insights into the application of chemotherapy in man. Following injection of a single cancer cell into an animal host, the development of tumor cells is described by an exponential growth curve. Each cell division doubles the number of cells. When 27 doublings have occurred, approximately one billion cancer cells are present. At this stage, the mass of the tumor is about one centimeter in diameter. Such a tumor in man would be barely detectable on chest roentgenogram in the case of lung cancer, or barely palpable as a breast mass. Even at this early stage, a vast number of cancer cells is present, so that even localized cancer at diagnosis is, in effect, "advanced" disease.

In patients with apparently localized and surgically resected tumor, micrometastases containing as few as 1000 cells may already exist in a distant site such as the lung or the liver, and these clusters are undetectable. Left untreated, they eventually develop into clinically evident metastatic disease, containing more than one trillion tumor cells per mass. Recurrence stems from undetectable micrometastatic disease that had been present initially. Thus, chemotherapy often is appropriate following excision of apparently localized disease in efforts to increase the potential for cure. One example is the use of cyclophosphamide-methotrexate-5-fluorouracil (CMF) chemotherapy in women with positive axillary nodes following mastectomy.

Chemotherapy is useful not only in attempts at cure but also in the palliation of advanced metastatic disease. In a patient with a measurable tumor mass (such as a palpable abdominal mass or pulmonary nodule that can be measured with calipers or a ruler), successful therapy can cause either a *complete response* (complete disappearance of all measurable and palpable tumor) or a *partial response* (a decrease of greater than 50% in the product of the largest perpendicular diameters of a tumor mass). Together, these responses define an objective response rate for a particular treatment. In general, patients who achieve a complete response with chemotherapy live significantly longer than those who achieve a partial response who, in turn, survive longer than non-responders. Patients achieving a complete or partial response generally have symptomatic relief far in excess of the toxicity of chemotherapy itself.

There are, of course, specific side effects of chemotherapy and these must be considered in assessing the cost/benefit ratio for the treatment of every patient. In conducting such an analysis, the clinician must address the following questions: is chemotherapy indicated; if so, what kind and how aggressive should it be; when should therapy be discontinued; what indeed are the risks; and what is the balance between side effects and the potential for benefit? Answers to these questions establish the relative risk/benefit ratio and determine whether and when treatment is appropriate.

If treatment is indicated medically, the next problem often is to motivate patients to accept it. This is especially problematic in light of chemotherapy's negative connotations. It may be helpful to view the success rate of cancer treatment relative to that of common non-malignant diseases. For example, chemotherapy for the most advanced stage of Hodgkin's disease cures 55% of patients,[2] whereas five-year survival, not even cure, of congestive heart failure secondary to hypertension in males is only 38%, as shown in the Framingham study.[3]

DEFINING SPECIFIC GOALS

Factors such as symptoms, age, ambulatory status, psychologic condition, economic circumstances, nutrition, and the specific site and extent of metastatic involvement must be considered in evaluating the individual patient. The administration of chemotherapy is not difficult. The dilemmas in chemotherapeutic treatment concern management decisions about when to give and when not to give drugs, when to suggest surgery or radiation therapy, or when all three modalities should be employed. It is necessary to work within the context of defining specific goals for the individual patient. Critical factors include a clear understanding of what needs to be accomplished for the patient and what the risk/benefit ratio is.

When the goal is cure, the level of acceptable risk can be quite high and a radical treatment plan involving aggressive and hazardous therapy may be warranted. For example, MOPP chemotherapy for advanced stages IIIB-IV Hodgkin's disease results in an 80% complete remission rate, and two-thirds of these patients are cured. Risks of life-threatening myelosuppression and opportunistic infections, in addition to hair loss, severe vomiting, neurologic toxicity, and male sterility attend this regimen. These risks are acceptable because no patient who fails to gain a complete remission will survive five years.[2]

Is the goal long-term palliation with significant prolongation of survival rather than cure? It is clear that patients who respond to chemotherapy, even those with disseminated metastatic disease, generally feel better and live longer than those who fail to respond. Long-term palliation provides additional months or years of life with concomitant relief of symptoms. It may be argued that additional survival at the cost of side effects is hardly worthwhile if the patient will die despite treatment. The additional time may be valuable to the patient, however, as it is to a mother with metastatic breast cancer whose teenage children need her presence and guidance, and to the person who wishes to see the birth of a grandchild. Such considerations enter the risk/benefit ratio. Most patients choose to accept some degree of side effects in return for a lengthened survival.

The major aim of therapy in advanced malignant disease is symptom relief and long-term palliation, just as it is for other illnesses such as diabetes or emphysema. The goals of medical oncology are similar to those of other medical subspecialties—to make the patient feel and function better and live longer if cure is impossible. When the goal is short-term palliation or relief of symptoms, the expectation is not prolongation of survival, but rather amelioration of specifc distressing problems such as pain, obstruction of a hollow viscus, or metabolic imbalance such as hypercalcemia. Short-term palliation is the therapeutic goal usually applied to the management of the terminally ill cancer patient.

At times, however, patients with advanced cancer may appear terminally ill, but, in fact, may have a tumor that is responsive to conventional or experimental chemotherapy. For example, a 62-year-old vigorous man with gastric carcinoma and lymphangitic pulmonary metastases appeared critically ill because of severe dyspnea. Institution of 5-fluorouracil-adriamycin-mitomycin (FAM combination) offered this patient a 40% chance of an objective remission with symptom relief, improvement of performance status, and prolongation of survival.[4]

There are several malignancies for which effective chemotherapy does not yet exist. One example is metastatic pancreatic cancer. Even when confronted with the fact that effective treatment is not available for this diagnosis, many patients persist in wanting something to be done, something attempted. If chemotherapy is given under these circumstances, there is always the hope for unexpected beneficial response. Most patients with cancer want and need that hope, and the physician must be responsive to it. Here, the goal of therapy is circumscribed and defined by the desires and needs of the patient.

Another important goal of cancer therapy lies within the framework of clinical research. We are continuously searching for more effective chemotherapeutic regimens. A clinical trial may be directed at determining which of two potentially effective therapies is superior in terms of response rates and prolongation of survival. Clinical research also may be directed, for example, at determining which of two equally effective drug regimens has the least acute and long-term toxic side effects. Clinical research also plays a useful role when no known effective therapy exists. The use of cis-platinum in combination with vinblastine and bleomycin for the treatment and cure of metastatic testicular cancer is an example of a major therapeutic advance whose efficacy was determined by clinical trials.

CHEMOTHERAPY FOR THE TERMINALLY ILL PATIENT: MANAGEMENT CONSIDERATIONS

When the intent of treatment is strictly palliation, the value of instituting chemotherapy must be weighed carefully. Table 4–1 lists some management considerations that enter into this decision. These factors should be considered in determining both the goals of chemotherapy and the means of accomplishing them for a particular patient. The integrated balance of these considerations influences the potential cost/benefit ratio of a proposed chemotherapy regimen more meaningfully than does the inherent effectiveness of the drugs themselves. Due regard for the multiple variables

TABLE 4–1. Management Considerations for the Use of Chemotherapeutic Agents in the Terminally Ill Patient.

Patient symptoms
Tempo of disease progression
Natural history of the specific tumor
Tumor responsiveness to chemotherapy
Age
Performance status
Nutrition
Concurrent medical problems
Psychologic status
Patient and family objectives
Quality of life
Toxicity of the proposed drug program

makes it easier to decide whether chemotherapy should be initiated.

Symptom relief is a major chemotherapeutic objective for the terminally ill patient. Patients with non-small-cell lung carcinoma and superior vena cava syndrome resistant to radiotherapy can benefit from combination chemotherapy for symptom relief. The use of prednisone to relieve air hunger from lymphangitic pulmonary metastases is another appropriate application of palliative chemotherapy. For example, a 52-year-old woman with metastatic gastric carcinoma was able to discard her oxygen, attend the wedding of her daughter, and function reasonably well for one month on prednisone.

The tempo of disease progression also is important in deciding whether chemotherapy should be initiated. The threat of a serious impending problem or concurrent oncologic emergency may dictate the necessity for chemotherapeutic intervention. Rapidly progressive disease frequently produces symptoms that are distressing to both the patient and the family. The decision here is whether the temporary reversal of the emergency situation can restore the patient to an adequate level of functioning with minimal side effects from the chemotherapy itself.

A 60-year-old painter with refractory chronic myelogenous leukemia and blast crisis developed a rapidly rising peripheral blast count of 120,000/mm^3. This patient was at high risk for intracranial leukostasis with secondary cerebral hemorrhagic infarction. In addition, his long bones were extremely tender and painful because of the burgeoning intramedullary leukemic cell population. The institution of oral hydroxyurea chemotherapy on an outpatient basis lowered the blast count, decreased the risk of cerebral hemorrhage, and relieved the bone pain. The risk/benefit ratio clearly favored the initiation of chemotherapy in this case.

Another example of chemotherapy's benefit for a terminally ill patient with an oncologic emergency is the treatment of hypercalcemia with low-dose intravenous mithramycin, which lowers serum calcium with little toxicity. A comatose hypercalcemic patient can thus be restored to clear mental status and can resume conversation with family and friends. However, there may come a time in the hypercalcemic patient's course when the decision is made to withhold mithramycin and to let the patient die peacefully. The decision to institute treatment clearly is not made on the basis of symptoms alone. Rather, it must include all of the factors listed above.

The natural history of the patient's specific tumor and whether that tumor type is responsive to conventional or experimental chemotherapy are also important considerations. A 37-year-old woman with alveolar soft part sarcoma had obliteration of pulmonary parenchyma by large metastases. The natural history of this tumor is one of slow progression. The patient's cancer had failed to respond to an adriamycin-containing combination regimen, to second-line chemotherapy with platinum, and to an investigational Phase II agent. Given the slow pace of the tumor and its demonstrated unresponsiveness to chemotherapy, no further treatment was recommended. She was spared the side effects of toxic drug programs that would not have benefited her.

The age of the patient may or may not be an appropriate factor in the physician's decision to administer chemotherapy. It is rare for a young adult with acute myelogenous leukemia refractory to all chemotherapeutic agents not to receive last-ditch treatment with a new Phase I or II drug. The patient may already be infected, jaundiced, cachectic, leukopenic, and thrombocytopenic, but it is an unusual physician who can resist even futile efforts to treat the young patient. Conversely, a 65-year-old man with newly diagnosed acute myelogenous leukemia may not be offered any aggressive chemotherapy aimed at complete remission because of his age. Yet elderly patients may well have as good a chance for initial remission and for prolonged survival as younger patients.[5] Such facts notwithstanding, advanced age is frequently a justifiable reason for withholding therapy and sparing the terminal patient toxicity for marginal gain.

The patient's performance status must be evaluated because it is a major determinant of both prognosis and tolerance to treat-

TABLE 4–2.   Eastern Cooperative Oncology Group Performance Status
Scale.

Grade	Description
0	Fully active, able to carry on all pre-disease activities without restriction.
1	Restricted in physically strenuous activity but ambulatory and able to carry out work of a light or sedentary nature.
2	Ambulatory and capable of all self-care but unable to carry out any work activities. Up and about 50% or more of waking hours.
3	Capable of only limited self-care, confined to bed or chair 50% or more of waking hours.
4	Completely disabled. Cannot carry on any self-care. Totally confined to bed or chair.

ment. Performance status is the clinician's observation of the overall appearance of a cancer patient, of how well the disease is tolerated, and, most importantly, of how the patient is functioning
on a daily basis. Table 4–2 describes the widely used Eastern
Cooperative Oncology Group performance status scale. Ambulatory patients have a performance status score of 0 to 1, while the
terminally ill patient, often significantly disabled by disease, has
a performance status of 3 to 4.

This assessment is important because poor performance status
has a negative prognostic impact on a patient's chances of responding to chemotherapy. For example, the objective response rate to
5-fluorouracil chemotherapy for metastatic colon carcinoma in a
patient with a performance status of 0 is 30%, whereas patients
with performance status of 3 or 4 exhibit less than 10% partial
response rate to the same drug. Because terminally ill patients
almost invariably have a performance status of 3 or 4, the role of
chemotherapy in these situations is inherently constricted.

The patient's nutritional status also affects response to chemotherapy. A 48-year-old man with pancreatic carcinoma and liver
metastases who has lost 25 pounds in the past two months and is
markedly cachectic and nauseated is not a candidate for chemotherapy. Administration of drugs to a patient in such a condition
would only further aggravate nausea and vomiting and hasten demise. Concurrent medical problems, such as severe congestive heart
failure, pulmonary disease, insulin-requiring diabetes mellitus, or
the presence of renal insufficiency also may limit the type and
intensity of chemotherapy appropriately applied and may contraindicate any treatment at all. Thus, empiric use of adriamycin cannot
be recommended in a patient with poorly controlled congestive

heart failure when the underlying tumor is not known to be responsive to this agent.

The psychologic status of the patient frequently affects the physician's judgment regarding chemotherapy in the terminally ill patient. It is a natural tendency to react negatively to the thought of administering chemotherapy to a severely depressed, withdrawn patient with far-advanced colon carcinoma. Conversely, one may be tempted to initiate an inappropriately aggressive chemotherapeutic regimen in a patient with the same disease who remains cheerful, hopeful, and apparently well-adjusted to the diagnosis.

The psychologic status of the patient is closely linked to the patient's objectives and to the expectations of what chemotherapy can hope to accomplish. In turn, the patient's outlook often is tied to and strongly influenced by the family's expectations, which may be unrealistic. The family's perspective may be inappropriately optimistic or pessimistic based on previous experiences with cancer or on media revelations of new "miracle" treatments. A major problem confronts the physician caught between the realities of a terminal illness and the unrealistic expectations of the patient or the family.

If the patient or family pressures the physician to treat and expects benefit from therapy when none can occur, it is best to strive to help the family gain a more realistic perspective. At times, however, it may be necessary to administer a relatively non-toxic chemotherapeutic agent to the patient who demands treatment in order to sustain hope without great expectation of benefit.

An example of this might be a woman whose metastatic breast carcinoma had responded previously to several different chemotherapeutic programs. Even in the terminal phase, her perspective may be that some other approach, as yet untried, might still be effective. She may be unwilling to accept a no-treatment option, and the physician may be persuaded to administer some form of chemotherapy with little expectation of benefit. The problem is more easily resolved if the patient is eligible for an investigational study of an experimental drug. The patient thus retains the hope that the disease will once again respond and can derive some sustenance from the knowledge that, at the least, future patients may be helped by her participation in the drug trial.

The physician should attend carefully to the patient's concerns and wishes after attempting to bring the patient and family to accept the fact of limited therapeutic options and end-stage disease.

Faced with the choice between no treatment or chemotherapy with mild or severe side effects, the patient should participate in the decision-making process. Candid and tactful discussion can result in a decision consonant with both the patient's needs and desires and the physician's best judgment.

Quality of life and normal tissue tolerance are important management considerations in terminal illness. Administration of chemotherapy can detract from the patient's ability to function in the last months of life and may impinge unacceptably on the patient's pride. Regrowth of hair once chemotherapy is stopped may be important to the patient. Withholding chemotherapy may allow a patient's limited marrow reserve to produce enough red and white cells and platelets to avoid the necessity for frequent blood component transfusions and hospitalizations for the management of infection.

For the majority of terminally ill patients, the side effects of chemotherapy do not warrant its application. This can be explained to the patient in an empathic manner and the patient can be brought to a level of acceptance. Many patients are relieved by the recommendation of no further chemotherapy.

Thus, chemotherapy for the terminally ill patient may be administered for the relief of symptoms, to meet the patient's need to sustain hope, or for clinical research purposes. Once treatment is initiated, the defined goals always should be kept in mind. Continuation of chemotherapy in the face of disease progression only enhances morbidity. Failure to alter therapy in the face of disease progression because the physician or family believes the patient "cannot tolerate more bad news" is not justifiable. For the physician and the patient, the decision not to use chemotherapy in terminally advanced, resistant disease is reached with difficulty, but it is usually correct.

REFERENCES

1. DeVita, V.T., Jr., Henney, J.E., and Stonehill, E.: Cancer mortality: the good news. *In:* Adjuvant Therapy of Cancer II. Edited by S.E. Jones, and S.E. Salmon. New York, Grune and Stratton, 1979, pp XV–XX.
2. DeVita, V.T., et al: Curability of advanced Hodgkin's disease with chemotherapy. Ann. Int. Med., *92*:587–595, 1980.
3. Kannel, W.B., et al: Role of blood pressure in the development of congestive heart failure: the Framingham study. N. Engl. J. Med., *287*:781–787, 1972.
4. Macdonald, J.S., et al: 5-Fluorouracil, doxorubicin, and mitomycin (FAM)

combination chemotherapy for advanced gastric cancer. Ann. Int. Med., *93*:533–536, 1980.

5. Foon, K.A., Zighelboim, J., Yale, C., and Gale, R.P.: Intensive chemotherapy is the treatment of choice for elderly patients with acute myelogenous leukemia. Blood, *58*:467–470, 1981.

Chapter 5

Palliative Radiation Therapy

Melvyn P. Richter

The chief aim of palliative radiotherapy is to alleviate distressing symptoms caused by incurable cancer. How successful the radiotherapy program is in achieving its goal in an individual patient depends on the extent of the disease, the functional status of the patient, and, to a lesser extent, the underlying histology. The patient's previous anti-cancer treatment is also a factor when considering a proposed course of palliative radiotherapy. For example, irradiation of extensive amounts of bone marrow in palliating multiple painful bone metastases is not possible in a patient who is leukopenic due to extensive prior chemotherapy or irradiation. Before a patient is approached with palliative intent it should be clearly determined that there is no potential for cure. In a patient with squamous cell carcinoma of the lung involving mediastinal lymph nodes, for example, cure by surgery may be unlikely and by irradiation less than 10%. The management team, therefore, may adopt a nihilistic approach to this patient, reserving therapy only for palliation of specific symptoms and signs. An individual with this type of tumor is still potentially curable, however, and should at least be offered the option of undergoing definitive therapy.

In all instances, the management team must document that the patient's symptoms are due to tumor before initiating palliative treatment. For example, not all chest pain in patients with cancer is related to the malignancy. Remediable, non-cancer-related problems do exist and deserve evaluation. Moreover, irradiating areas in a cancer patient on the assumption that tumor is located there

TABLE 5–1. General Principles of Palliative Therapy.

1. Establish that the disease is beyond cure.
2. Determine that tumor is in fact the cause of the symptoms.
3. Establish realistic treatment goals.
    a. Should the patient be treated at all?
    b. What approach can the patient best tolerate?
4. Establish clear communication among members of the treatment team and with the patient.
5. Start with the least morbid effective therapies.
6. Avoid producing debilitating side effects that are worse than the symptoms being treated for palliation.

can cause unneeded problems. In most instances, the clinician should document that tumor masses are present in symptomatic regions before treating the patient. To what length this diagnostic evaluation is pursued depends greatly upon the experience of the clinicians making the evaluation. Balanced against the need for definitive diagnosis is the fact that untimely delay of effective, specific management directed toward a cancer-related symptom may create unnecessary suffering for the patient (Table 5–1).

The availability of different specialists strongly influences which palliative maneuver is selected. Radiation therapists are most effective when they function as part of a management team consisting of specialists in chemotherapy, radiation therapy, surgery and its subspecialties, anesthesiology, rehabilitation medicine, social service, and psychosocial and nutritional support.

COMMON USES OF PALLIATIVE RADIOTHERAPY

Table 5–2 lists the radiotherapy consultations performed at the Fox Chase Cancer Center in 1980 according to primary site and type of therapy offered (curative, palliative, or no radiation treatment). An individual patient may have undergone multiple consultations during the course of the year. Lung cancer, including all histologic types, is invariably the predominant tumor seen by radiation therapists. After lung cancer, the most frequent tumors seen by radiotherapists for palliation are cancers of the breast, genitourinary and gastrointestinal tracts, head and neck, gynecologic malignancies, and lymphatic system (mainly non-Hodgkin's lymphoma).

Listed below are cancer diagnoses and specific problems for which palliative radiation therapy consultation is sought:

Cancer Diagnosis	Common Problems Amenable to Palliative Radiotherapy
1. Lung Cancer	Airway obstruction Vascular and esophageal compression Hemoptysis Tumor-induced chest and bone pain Brain metastases
2. Breast Cancer	Bone metastases Chest wall recurrence Central nervous system metastases Inoperable breast cancer
3. Genitourinary Cancer	Painful skeletal metastases (prostate) Urinary hemorrhage or obstruction
4. Gastrointestinal Cancer	Esophageal obstruction (gastric and esophageal cancer) Pelvic and perineal pain (recurrent rectal carcinoma) Distant metastases to bone and brain Painful hepatic invasion
5. Carcinoma of the Head and Neck	Reduction of tumor bulk Control of bleeding and infection Pain relief
6. Gynecologic Malignancies	Control of hemorrhage Lymphatic ureteral obstruction Pelvic pain

The application of palliative irradiation is based on consideration of the following factors:

1. The availability of radiotherapeutic facilities and trained personnel.
2. The overall time required for the patient to receive the radiotherapy program.
3. The patient's previous chemotherapy and irradiation.
4. The radiation tolerance of normal tissues within the radiation field.
5. Technical radiation therapy factors such as total dose, treatment volume, energy of radiation (orthovoltage versus megavoltage), and portal design.
6. The overall management of the patient's needs rather than the resolution of a single problem.

Palliative radiotherapy may be administered either by a short course of irradiation delivered with individual fractions greater

TABLE 5–2.   Results of Radiation Therapy Consultations (N = 1216 Patients).*

Site	% of Total Patients Seen	Therapy Decisions Curative (No.)	Palliative (No.)	No XRT† (No.)
Lung	25	80	180	45
Breast	14	40	100	28
G.U.	10	45	60	19
G.I.	10	35	56	27
Head & neck	9	64	29	21
GYN	8	56	9	29
Skin cancer:				
Melanoma	2	—	16	7
Other	5	46	3	9
Lymphoma:				
Hodgkin's	2	20	2	3
Non-Hodgkin's	4	17	20	8
CNS	3	26	6	5
Miscellaneous	9	27	51	27
		456	532	228

*American Oncologic Hospital, 1980.
†No radiation therapy.

than 200 rad, typically over a period of less than 2 weeks, or by a more protracted course delivered with conventional fractions of 200 rad or less over a longer period of time.

A short course of irradiation may be appropriate in patients with the following conditions:

1. Rapid tumor progression.
2. Early dissemination following definitive treatment.
3. Short life expectancy (less than 3 months).

Examples of short treatment courses include the following:

1. 1000 rad in 1 fraction for a painful metastasis to bone that is not in danger of pathologic fracture.
2. 2000 rad in 5 fractions over 1 week or 3000 rad in 10 fractions over 2 weeks for the majority of axial skeleton metastases or brain metastases.

A protracted course of irradiation may be appropriate in a patient with the following conditions:

1. An anticipated life expectancy greater than 3 months.
2. Indolent disease.
3. Large tumor masses (i.e., greater than 10 × 10 cm).
4. A solitary metastasis where the primary tumor is controlled.
5. Locally extensive tumors of the head and neck, genitourinary or female reproductive systems, where effective palliative radiation doses approach the curative doses. Doses of 4000 to 5000 rad over 3 to 6 weeks usually provide palliation in such instances.

Potential damage to normal tissues within the radiation therapy field is a factor in determining the maximum total dose and the individual daily radiation dose that can be utilized. There is a substantial body of data defining the normal tissue tolerance of critical organs such as brain, spinal cord, heart, bowel, liver, kidney, lung, and skin.[1] In a short course of irradiation, using large individual fractions (>400 rads), immediate radiation effects on normal tissues may not be apparent. However, should the patient enjoy a significant survival time (i.e., beyond six months), the delayed effects of radiation may appear with fibrosis and vascular damage causing impaired function and disability. In irradiating large areas of the abdomen, as in the palliation of a mesenteric lymphoma and gastric or pancreatic carcinoma, it is often necessary to irradiate one kidney. The management team must first establish that adequate bilateral renal function exists to compensate for the eventual loss of the irradiated kidney.

BONE METASTASES

The management of painful bone metastases is the palliative problem most frequently seen by radiation therapists. Lung, breast, and prostate cancers comprise the majority of the cases. Approximately 70% of all patients experience some pain relief at 4 weeks following radiotherapy.[2] Improved results were reported by Ambrad,[3] at the Philadelphia Veterans Administration Hospital, who utilized a *short course* of irradiation with *large individual fractions*. Almost all patients reported some degree of improvement by the second week and most were completely free of pain by the fourth week, with prolonged pain relief persisting over the median survival of five months. An argument in favor of rapid palliation, especially in terminally ill cancer patients, is that less time is spent by the patient in a radiotherapy facility. For the spine or skull, 2000 rad in 1 week in 5 equal fractions represents a reasonable compromise between speed and tolerance.

For the long bones, the issue may not be pain relief alone. Where the structural integrity of the bone is preserved, there is generally no need for internal fixation. Some radiation therapists feel, however, that higher total doses administered in daily fractions of 200 to 300 rad are more likely to produce healing or at least to prevent progression of lytic or blastic disease at the treated site.

Where fracture is evident or imminent, palliative radiotherapy, for the most part, should be avoided unless combined with internal fixation. Radiation alone prevents callus formation without some form of internal mechanical stabilization.[4] It is recommended, therefore, for individuals with survival times estimated to be greater than one month, that surgery be performed utilizing either metal internal fixation devices or prostheses fixed in place with methyl methacrylate.[5] Following these orthopedic procedures, it may be unnecessary to offer immediate palliative radiotherapy to the region unless there is persistent pain or extensive osseous and soft tissue involvement. There is no contraindication to administering the irradiation preoperatively.

BRAIN METASTASES

Brain metastases require prompt management. Seizures and headache, resulting from increased intracranial pressure, can be completely relieved by palliative cranial irradiation delivered by various treatment schedules. Results from a group-wide experience show an overall response rate of approximately 60% with median survival of 4 to 6 months.[6] Ambulatory patients tend to survive longer than those who are non-ambulatory. In cancer patients with brain metastases and good performance status, tumor type affects prognosis. Thus, patients with breast cancer survive longer (21 weeks median) than do those with lung cancer (12 weeks median).

In patients with a solitary metastasis or good functional status, there may be an advantage in utilizing total doses greater than 2000 rad in 1 week or 3000 rad over 2 to 3 weeks. This may be accomplished by reducing the radiation treatment volume to the known gross disease for an additional boost or by continuing the whole brain irradiation program to 4000 to 5000 rad. In surgically accessible solitary brain metastases from malignant melanoma or renal cell carcinoma, excision followed by whole brain radiation produces the most effective palliation.

In symptomatic patients, corticosteroid therapy (dexamethasone, 16 mg/day in divided dosage) should be instituted immediately because it produces a more rapid response than radiotherapy by immediately reducing edema. With corticosteroids, even symptomatic patients may demonstrate improved functional status sufficient to permit outpatient radiation therapy. The corticosteroid response alone, however, is not durable unless radiotherapy is administered. Continued symptomatic improvement after initiation of radiotherapy may permit discontinuation of corticosteroids to avoid potential side effects of long-term therapy.

SPINAL CORD COMPRESSION

Approximately 5% of cancer patients develop spinal epidural metastases. Most commonly, the epidural deposits represent local extension from metastatic tumor involving the vertebrae. Severe or persistent back pain, unexplained constipation or urinary difficulty, or other neurologic changes should alert the clinician to this possibility. Evaluation should not be delayed and includes appropriate radiographs, myelogram, and spinal fluid analysis. If an epidural block is demonstrated, the clinician must define the extent of the compression above and below the obstruction to define precisely the boundaries of the regional irradiation portal.

Laminectomy may be in order to establish the diagnosis in patients presenting without a previously known cancer. In all other instances, however, the role of decompressive laminectomy is unclear. Surgery alone has been demonstrated to be inferior to a combination of surgery with irradiation and to radiation alone.[7] The issue of when to utilize surgical decompression with irradiation is currently under active investigation. It is generally agreed, however, that for patients with widely metastatic bronchogenic carcinoma, which is the most common cause of epidural spinal cord compression, there is no benefit to surgical decompression.

As with symptomatic intracranial metastases, corticosteroids should be used to decrease the spinal cord edema produced by the epidural metastasis. Full doses should be maintained throughout the course of therapy and tapered as appropriate following completion of radiotherapy. Most cancer centers have adopted initial radiotherapy fractions of higher than 200 rad to produce rapid tumor cell kill and to decrease inflammatory response. After 3 individual daily fractions of 400 rad, fraction sizes of 180 to 200 rad are utilized to total doses of approximately 3000 to 3600 rad.

For radiation-responsive tumors such as lymphoma, the lower total dose is appropriate. For the majority of solid tumors, however, the higher dose is employed. For those individuals who do not have significant neurologic deficit at the time of initiation of therapy, it is reasonable to use conventional fractionation and shrinking field technique, carrying therapy to the lesion up to the spinal cord tolerance of approximately 4000 to 4400 rad.

The clinical response is directly related to the degree of functional impairment antedating the initiation of therapy. Patients presenting with paraplegia and no bladder and bowel function for more than 24 hours rarely improve sufficiently to regain ambulation. On the other hand, approximately 60% of patients who are ambulatory at the time of the diagnosis of cord compression remain so after treatment, and one third of those with mild to moderate weakness can be converted to an ambulatory state. In general, the more rapid the onset and progression of the neurologic findings, the worse the prognosis, as compared with that for patients with a longer history of evolving neurologic deficits.[7]

MENINGEAL METASTASES

The common cancers that spread to the meninges are breast cancer, non-Hodgkin's lymphoma, and acute leukemia. Unlike the hematologic cancers, meningeal metastases from solid tumors such as breast cancer occur only with terminal illness. The symptoms are similar to those of brain metastases but most patients also show multifocal findings and cranial nerve palsies. Diagnostic evaluation is discussed in Chapter 3.

Therapy usually consists of a combination of intrathecal methotrexate and palliative radiotherapy to the whole brain. Because of the discomfort of repeated lumbar punctures for intrathecal therapy and because this route does not ensure adequate delivery of methotrexate to higher levels of the neuraxis, an Ommaya reservoir may be implanted beneath the scalp. This permits ready access to the ventricular spinal fluid by subcutaneous puncture. However, in carcinomatous meningitis, there are often nodular deposits of tumor throughout the neuraxis (as opposed to the sheets of cells in leukemic and lymphomatous meningitis), which hamper effective drug penetration of tumor cells. An alternative therapy is craniospinal radiation without intrathecal chemotherapy, but this is associated with increased morbidity.

How vigorously to approach this problem depends on the global status of the patient and the disease. Approximately 50% of patients improve symptomatically for periods of 2 to 5 months. High-dose corticosteroids are also helpful here. In a patient near death for reasons independent of meningeal metastases, treatment with corticosteroids alone is the appropriate treatment option.

HEMORRHAGE AND OBSTRUCTION

Massive bleeding produced by tumor erosion of a blood vessel does not benefit from emergency irradiation. Interventional angiography with selective catheterization and infarction of the bleeding vessel(s) yields more immediate results. Palliative radiotherapy can be effective in controlling moderate hematemesis from esophageal or gastric carcinoma. Irradiation produces reduction in tumor bulk, thereby promoting healing through re-epithelialization and scar formation.

Hemorrhage is often a major component of advanced pelvic neoplasms, such as squamous cell carcinoma of the cervix and adenocarcinoma of the endometrium. Intravaginal cone irradiation or limited pelvic external irradiation utilizing an abbreviated course of 1000 to 1500 rad often produces hemostasis. Less predictable results are seen in recurrent adenocarcinoma of the rectum and sigmoid colon, in regionally advanced transitional cell carcinoma of the bladder, and in adenocarcinoma of the prostate.

Pelvic and referred pain and ureteral obstruction generally require whole pelvis radiotherapy to total doses of 4000 to 5000 rad by shrinking field technique in which the irradiated volume is gradually reduced in size, focusing down upon the gross tumor volume. Complete obstruction of the urinary and fecal stream rarely is relieved by palliative radiotherapy except in the case of lymphomas. In such cases, limited surgical intervention is effective and humane. It can improve quality of life in individuals who otherwise enjoy good functional status and who have a reasonable likelihood of surviving longer than days or weeks.

THORACIC PROBLEMS IN LUNG CANCER

The management of airway obstruction, hemoptysis, chest pain, and shortness of breath caused by lung cancer of all histologic types is a major palliative concern. Relief of such symptoms by radiation therapy does not extend survival but clearly improves its quality. Wherever feasible, irradiated lung volume should be restricted to exclude as much noninvolved lung as possible, in order to reduce the risk and extent of radiation-induced pulmonary fibrosis and pneumonitis. In the presence of widespread disease, there is no reason to use doses of irradiation employed for cure, namely, 5000 rad or greater. Radiotherapy usually is successful in controlling hemoptysis, relieving airway obstruction, and alleviating the deep intrathoracic pain that is commonly experienced by these patients. Rarely does irradiation cause reversal of phrenic nerve and recurrent laryngeal nerve palsy from tumor.

Obstruction of venous return, the classic superior vena caval syndrome, can be improved in the majority of patients with irradiation directed at the thoracic inlet and mediastinum. When short course, high individual radiation dose programs are used, care must be taken to consider the normal tissue tolerances of spinal cord and heart. This is particularly important in patients previously or concurrently treated with adriamycin, which is itself cardiotoxic and can enhance the radiation reaction.

An integrated effort of medical and paramedical specialists can produce efficient and humane management of patients with incurable cancer so that an acceptable quality of life is achieved. At least, the management team should seek the alleviation of severe pain. New techniques of palliative radiotherapy employing short courses minimize the burdens of therapy. In many cases, improved function results in a concomitant reduction in inpatient hospital care. The development of hospice programs and the increasing sensitivity of the medical team to the social, psychologic, and economic consequences of incurable cancer permit an integrated analysis and effective application of the principles of palliative care.

REFERENCES

1. Vaeth, J.M. (ed): Frontiers of Radiation Therapy and Oncology, Vol. 6, Radiation Effects and Tolerance, Normal Tissue. Baltimore, University Park Press, 1972.
2. Hendricksen, F.R., and Pagano, M.: Palliation of osseous metastases: preliminary report. In Bone Metastasis. Edited by L. Weiss, and H.A. Gilbert. Boston, G.K. Hall, 1981.
3. Ambrad, A.: Single dose and short high-dose fractionation radiation therapy for osseous metastases. In Bone Metastasis. Edited by L. Weiss, and H.A. Gilbert. Boston, G.K. Hall, 1981.
4. Bonarigo, B., and Rubin, P.: Nonunion of pathologic fracture after radiation therapy. Radiology, 88:889–898, 1967.
5. Harrington, K.D.: The management of malignant pathologic fractures. In

Bone Metastasis. Edited by L. Weiss, and H.A. Gilbert. Boston, G.K. Hall, 1981.

6. Borget, B., et al: The palliation of brain metastases: final results of the first two studies by the Radiation Therapy Oncology Group. Int. J. Radiat. Oncol. Biol. Phys., *6*:1–9, 1980.

7. Black, P.: Metastatic tumors of the central nervous system: spinal metastases. *In* Complications of Cancer, Diagnosis and Management. Edited by M. Abeloff. Baltimore, Johns Hopkins University Press, 1979.

Chapter 6

Psychophysiology of Pain

Janet L. Abrahm

Chapter 17 of this book provides specific treatment guidelines for the range of symptoms that cancer patients experience. This chapter deals with the evaluation of and various therapeutic approaches to one common symptom, that of pain. Pain is experienced or feared by a majority of cancer patients. During the last decade, major studies have focused on ways of conceptualizing, treating, and exploring the meaning of pain in cancer patients and on understanding what it does to their families. The hospice movement has contributed importantly to increased understanding and ability to manage pain successfully. Our approach to the evaluation of pain includes attention not only to *what* is hurting, but also to *why* it is hurting so much. Various treatment strategies are outlined for application either alone or in combination.

PATHOPHYSIOLOGY OF PAIN

The pathophysiology of the actual sensation and experience of pain is not entirely clear. No nerve has been found that, when stimulated, always produces reliable reports of pain. This is true even for stimuli that might be assumed to be invariably painful, such as sensations associated with tooth extraction. For example, children who have not been taught that dental extractions are supposed to be frightening and painful report sensations during extraction, but these sensations would not necessarily be defined as pain. In the absence of definitive understanding of pathophysiology, several theories of pain perception have been advanced.[1-3]

Afferent nerves carry reports of nerve-ending stimulation. The nerve endings are specialized receptors that trigger impulses in response to temperature change, touch, pressure, and noxious stimuli. Information from the nerves, transmitted through afferent pathways in the spinal cord, ascends through spinothalamic tracts to the thalamus and then to the cortex. Conscious perception of the stimulus then occurs.

The gate theory of Melzack and Wall proposes that a specific nerve cell in the spinal cord, the "T cell," responds to both excitatory and inhibitory impulses, the summation of which determines whether the nerve will fire.[1] Afferent nerve input to the T cell is modulated in the substantia gelatinosa. In addition, descending inhibitory pathways from the brain modulate the firing of the spinal cord T cell. Thus, a "gate" is hypothesized through which afferent nerve impulses must pass before being relayed to the brain. Whether the "gate" is open or closed is determined by factors other than a simple sum of the afferent impulses. This theory proposes that the complexity of the experience of pain is explained by these modifying factors.

One major problem with this theory is that the T cell has not been identified. There is also a lack of precise, one-to-one correspondence between specific spinal cord areas and the sensation of pain in a particular part of the body. The lack of precise knowledge about specific fibers that transmit the sensation of pain hampers our ability to treat it. Pain perception is a complex event involving afferent stimuli to the cord, descending inhibitory impulses to the cord, and multiple modifying influences operative at the thalamic and cortical levels of the brain.

Weisenberg's conceptualization, that pain is a psychologic experience,[4] encompasses the complexity of relevant factors more thoroughly than do alternate hypotheses. Although physiologic correlates of the psychologic experience of pain exist, pain differs fundamentally from other sensory experiences such as touch, color vision, or hearing. One major difference is that objective evidence of the intensity of noxious stimuli does not correspond with the extent of pain experienced by the individual.

SITUATIONAL COMPONENTS OF RESPONSE TO PAIN

Montaigne eloquently noted, "We feel one cut from the surgeon's scalpel more than ten blows of the sword in the heat of battle." Beecher, an army surgeon, documented that the degree of pain reported, and the subsequent amount of analgesia needed, failed to correlate with the extent of injury, but varied instead with the setting and significance of the wound.[5,6] In treating wounded soldiers who had survived the beach assault on Anzio during the Second World War, he found that minimal or no analgesic medication was required. These same soldiers complained loudly about the pain of an inept venipuncture attempt, but much less so about wound pain, which meant a ticket home. When Dr. Beecher later saw similar injuries in his civilian practice, he found that substantially more analgesia was required than had been needed in his Army hospital experience. For the civilians, injuries and surgery meant disruption of their usual lives and routines, loss of income, and impeded normal function. For the soldiers, on the other hand, the injuries represented the opportunity to return to their homes and to normal existence, and an escape from war and its hazards.

PSYCHOLOGIC COMPONENTS OF RESPONSE TO PAIN

Whatever the precise neural pathways of pain, a broad array of psychic responses greatly influences its perception. Pain is differently perceived on the basis of its site and cause. It is interpreted variously, depending on the patient's circumstances, emotional and physical condition, and psychologic coping mechanisms. Pain can imply danger, physical damage, fear, anxiety, or punishment. It can suggest also a need to obtain or avoid treatment, and it may serve as a means of judging the effectiveness of treatment. Pain may increase in severity when it loses meaning, such as occurs in the chronic pain often experienced by the terminal cancer patient.

Chapman explores the ramifications of patients' emotional status in an effort to uncover the dynamics of the pain experience.[7] He demonstrates how fear of loss of physical ability, fear of disfigurement, a sense of helplessness, and the impact of financial problems all lead to depression. Depression amplifies the perception of noxious stimuli, as does anger resulting from resentment of sickness and therapeutic failure. Fear of uncontrollable pain, fear of loss of social position or self control, and fear of death also lead to considerable anxiety which similarly modifies bodily signals and how they are interpreted. The general physical condition of the patient and the stage of medical care (diagnosis, active therapy, palliative therapy, no therapy) also contribute to how patients perceive and modulate discomfort.

CULTURAL COMPONENTS OF RESPONSE TO PAIN

The degree to which patients complain about pain is also modified by cultural factors. Several studies support the not surprising notion that various ethnic groups react differently to pain.[8] One's rearing and one's learned, culturally accepted modes of dealing with painful stimuli affect not only one's perception of noxious stimuli, but also the style and amplitude of one's expression of pain. If the individual's upbringing favored stoicism, pain response may be muted. If tacit approval was given to expressive emotional response to any noxious stimulus in childhood, pain tolerance in adulthood may be reduced and an emotive response would be the conditioned reaction.[9]

DURATION OF THE PAIN EXPERIENCE

The duration and severity of pain also influence response to it. Chronic and acute pain evoke different physiologic reactions to the same noxious stimulus. All of the problems faced in coping with acute pain are magnified in the chronic pain situation. While experiencing chronic pain, the individual must continue to deal with day-to-day events and with the ongoing obligations and problems of existence, such as finances and interpersonal stresses. The longer the pain persists, the longer one is denied the time and opportunity to deal with it. The constellation of personal relationships and emotional responses to them, as well as the perception of self, are altered by the continuous presence of pain.

THE CAUSE OF PAIN IN THE CANCER PATIENT

Bonica's summary article on cancer pain reports that 75% of pain experienced was caused by the cancer itself;[10] 20% by the therapy; and, importantly, 5% was incidental, that is, entirely unrelated to the cancer. This finding underscores the importance of evaluating each new pain to isolate its cause. The automatic assumption that any new pain can be attributed to the cancer is unwarranted. Therapeutic response to pain depends on its etiology and relationship to the disease.

The actual frequency of non-cancer pain perceived by patients is much higher than the 5% reported. The patient generally perceives any ache or pain, such as a sore back or a headache, as cancer-related. Every pain should be investigated for its etiology lest inappropriate therapy be administered.

THE MANAGEMENT OF PAIN: CONVENTIONAL APPROACHES AND PROBLEMS

Treatment of the Tumor

Because 75% of pain in cancer patients is tumor-related, every attempt should be made to alleviate the pain by directly treating the malignancy itself. Surgery directed at tumor removal or at relief of tumor-caused obstruction, radiation therapy, chemotherapy, or hormonal therapy can afford much relief even when cure is not possible.

Pharmacologic Approaches

When initiating pharmacologic treatment for pain, the physician generally uses non-narcotic analgesics such as aspirin or acetaminophen. These drugs frequently are effective, and their utility may be enhanced by the concomitant administration of non-analgesic medication such as diazepam for relief of secondary painful muscle spasm or non-steroidal anti-inflammatory agents such as phenylbutazone (Butazolidin) and ibuprofen for relief of secondary inflammatory response.

When narcotic analgesia is required, the guiding principles are the following: (1) administer medication in dosages sufficient to relieve the pain; (2) give it often enough to keep the patient comfortable; (3) use the most convenient dosage form (usually oral); and (4) reassure the patient that you will continue to monitor the pain and that the pain will be relieved.

The major problem in applying these precepts for physicians, nurses, and patients arises from a prevalent misunderstanding of the distinction between physical dependence and addiction. Physical dependence is a biochemical and/or physiologic adaptation of tissues, whereby continued administration of the agent becomes necessary for normal function. Tolerance is a gradual development of resistance to the effects of the drug upon repeated administration, wherein escalating dosages are required to maintain the desired effect. Tolerance and physical dependence typically occur to some degree.

Addiction, on the other hand, connotes drug-seeking behavior with goals other than that of pain relief. It is the negative implication of narcotic use that frequently stymies attempts to achieve effective pain control. Unfortunately, the term "addiction" is used at times also to signify physical dependence.

Maintaining a careful distinction between these terms—physical dependence and addiction—prevents confusion and establishes a useful therapeutic perspective. There is nothing inherently wrong with relieving pain and creating physical dependence on a drug if that is medically required. Research has indicated repeatedly that achieving pain relief for cancer patients does not induce addiction.[11,12] In fact, administering medication in amounts adequate to provide pain relief actually prevents establishing a cycle of drug-seeking behavior. When the objectives of pain elimination are achieved, the patient is not obliged to manipulate anyone in order to obtain narcotics. The cycle of experiencing pain, seeking relief, and coercing someone to provide narcotics is broken.

Patients who are physically dependent on narcotics can be tapered off when the pain remits.[13,14] They then become physically independent of the drugs. Unfortunately, the medical community has been slow to recognize this fact. Studies document that pain medication often is ordered incorrectly by physicians, and that nurses fail to give the full amount prescribed.[11] There is a persistent reluctance to provide adequate pain relief.

Educating the patient about any narcotic prescription is necessary in order to ensure compliance and achieve pain relief, especially when many patients have inappropriate fears of addiction. The physician must assume that some mythology and misconceptions exist for the patient, and must act tactfully to dispel them. By engaging honestly in discussion and providing reassurance, the physician can block feelings of guilt, eliminate a sense of inadequacy, and dispel fears. Patients can be taught that narcotic medication taken properly can provide the pain control necessary to a productive existence. Families as well as patients require careful explanations, often more than once, about the approach to pain relief. Such explanations provide substantial comfort for families and increase the likelihood that the patient will adhere to the needed regimen.

Drug Schedules

To use analgesic medications properly, the physician must know about the drugs, their side effects, duration of action, metabolism and excretion, and most effective means of administration. Meperidine (Demerol) is an inappropriate drug for chronic pain and should not be used. Its half-life is too short, and the side effects of effective doses are too great. Morphine, oxycodone, and methadone are often the mainstays of pain therapy, although other drugs, such as dihydromorphinone (Dilaudid), also are useful. It is best to select two or three drugs, know them well, and use them.

Tricyclic antidepressants often enhance the efficacy of narcotic analgesics and help reduce the amount of narcotic required for pain relief. The overall aim is to maximize pain relief and minimize side effects. If patients are best served by sleeping much of the time, or if they need to be awake during certain periods of the day, regimens can be modified to achieve these aims. The usual approach to narcotic administration in cancer patients involves gaining control of the pain by escalating dosages as frequently as possible in the first few days of therapy. Oral medication should be used if possible, or parenteral medication may be instituted initially for pain control with a view toward later implementation of equivalent oral dosage. The approach is similar to adjusting heparin dosage for anticoagulation by careful monitoring of the response to treatment.

Unfortunately, there is no simple blood test to measure analgesic response. Continued assessment on the basis of the patient's own reactions and perceptions of comfort will guide escalation of doses or addition of new medication. A short hospitalization is useful to adjust the regimen. This can be accomplished at home as well, but it is often frightening for the family because the drugs may be altered frequently. Drug schedules and side effects are detailed in Chapter 17.

NEUROSURGICAL APPROACHES TO PAIN

Neurosurgical approaches to pain involve impairing the pathway of noxious stimuli to the brain,[10] or eliminating those cortical centers that process the information. This approach is sometimes limited because pain fibers associated with the area of cancer-induced pain cannot always be located and/or transected with any specificity. Diagnostic or therapeutic nerve blocks may be helpful.[15-17] Local anesthesia of peripheral sensory nerves can identify appropriate patients for peripheral nerve damage. Chemicals, such as alcohol, can be injected to destroy sensory nerves. This can be effective, as the nerve may not regenerate for some time.

Ablative neurosurgical procedures are sometimes useful.[18-23] Sensory nerves can be cut at any level as they enter the spinal cord, although the problem of nerve regeneration exists. Rhizotomy is reasonable at times but requires resection of roots at multiple levels of the cord, because sensory nerves from one area enter the cord at different levels. Cutting the ascending spinothalamic (pain sensory) tract may also be effective if done at multiple cord levels. Unfortunately, pain persists in 25% or more of those who have undergone extensive neurosurgical resection. In half of patients who are treated neurosurgically, excellent pain relief is achieved. However, the usual side effects include distressingly large areas of local anesthesia or dysesthesia and incidental motor fiber transection with loss of function, which many patients find unacceptable.

The gate control theory suggests that descending nerve fibers suppress pain transmission. Electrical stimulation of these fibers may enhance their activity to the patient's benefit.[24,25] The stimulation can be controlled by the patient. The electrodes can be used superficially or implanted internally in peripheral sites or in the brain. Such invasive procedures are withheld until other alternatives have been exhausted.

MODIFICATION OF PSYCHOLOGIC RESPONSE TO PAIN

The patient's general psychologic status contributes significantly to pain perception, as discussed earlier in this chapter. Depression commonly accompanies chronic pain. Antidepressant medication modifies the patient's level of response to pain and pain tolerance, and special intervention may be sought to help patients with other problem areas of life. Through psychotherapy, religious counseling, financial counseling, and the use of interpersonal support structures, stress—caused by the cancer or not—may be ameliorated.

HYPNOSIS

Hypnosis can be valuable in modifying pain perception in patients with chronic cancer pain, and its application addresses many relevant psychologic issues as well. Kroger reviews the historical development of hypnosis and its application.[26,33] In ancient times, Aesculapius and his followers, in their healing temples, utilized a hypnosis-like approach to their patients. Mesmer, one of the first to use what we now call hypnosis, entered in flowing purple robes amid a number of sufferers as they sat in a vat of water, holding onto iron rods. He convinced patients that he could harness healing magnetic forces from the universe. Patients, in fact, were "mesmerized," and some of them were healed.

Elliotson and Esdaile, British surgeons who had heard of Mesmer's work, believed that mental power could be applied against pain. Esdaile performed thousands of operations in India with no anesthesia other than hypnosis and with convincing results,[27] but he was ridiculed when he returned to England. Braid, a Scottish physician contemporary with Esdaile, coined the term "hypnosis," meaning sleep-like state, later discovering that sleep is not involved in the phenomenon.

Hypnosis was promoted in France by Liebeault, a country doctor, and Bernheim, a renowned neurologist, in the second half of the nineteenth century. They also introduced the concepts of suggestion and suggestability, and considered hypnosis to be a function of normal behavior.[26] Freud studied with Bernheim and learned the technique of inducing trance. When Freud found that he did not need trance in order to communicate effectively, he abandoned hypnosis. Rasputin may have used hypnosis to stop the bleeding of the hemophiliac son of the czar of Russia.

Recently, a revival in enthusiasm for hypnosis has occurred, probably because of increasing interest in self-care. The teaching of hypnosis for medical and dental purposes has been accredited both in England (in 1955) and the United States (in 1958) as a safe, effective procedure.

Definitions

Terms that have specialized meanings when applied to discussions of hypnosis are defined below.[28] A hypnotic *trance* is a state of altered awareness in which communication between the patient and the hypnotist is facilitated. *Induction* is the method used to help attain the hypnotic state. The hypnotist does not induce a trance, but rather assists the patient to experience one. If the trance is self-induced by the patient, this is called *self hypnosis;* trance induced by the hypnotist is *heterohypnosis*. A *suggestion* is an idea that is so presented that it is accepted by the patient with a minimum of analysis, criticism, and resistance. *Dissociation* indicates splitting of perception of one part of the body or personality from another. *Distraction* is a diversion of attention. *Negative hallucination* eliminates the perception of something that objectively is present. For example, if one is in a trance, the suggestion can be made that a loudly flapping window shade will not be heard. *Positive hallucinations* can be auditory, visual, tactile, and so on. They establish the presence of something that is not really there. Any or all of these modes may be helpful in blocking pain perception, as described below.

Popular misconceptions about hypnosis abound. Used for medical or dental purposes, hypnosis is not an amusement but a therapeutic technique. Patients in a trance are not asleep. Their eyes may be closed or open, and they can be walking or sitting comfortably. Hypnosis itself is not a therapy. Therapy (e.g., pain relief) can take place while the patient is in trance. The hypnotist teaches the patient how to experience a state of trance, and may give helpful suggestions while the person is in the trance. The hypnotic state itself facilitates the giving and receiving of suggestions relative to the specific goals involved.

No one can be made to enter a trance unwillingly, and what occurs during the trance is entirely up to the subject. Nothing can be done that violates the individual's moral or ethical beliefs. People exit from trance whenever they desire.

The spontaneous induction of a trance-like state occurs frequently as a natural phenomenon. An athlete's "playing through the pain" is one example; another occurs at the theater, when one is so engrossed in the play that surrounding activity is ignored. Removing oneself from painful or difficult situations is an automatic, inherent survival technique.

Approximately 5 to 10% of the population cannot experience trance to any degree. Most people, however, are able to enter a trance state adequate to provide benefit. About 10% of people are capable of undergoing surgery with trance as the only anesthetic.[29,30] Differences in degrees of suggestability, which can be assessed, affect what can be accomplished by hypnosis.[29–31]

Clinically, ability to benefit from trance depends on the degree of motivation; the patient has to *want* to use trance to solve a problem, such as pain. In general, individuals with a good work history, many friends, good family relationships and leisure activities, who are creative and not severely depressed tend to make the best subjects. However, even severely depressed people can benefit if they are well motivated.

Communication with the trance subject can be verbal or totally nonverbal, involving gestures alone. Thus, dentists who work with deaf patients, through the use of visual cues, are able to obtain anesthesia in the jaw.[32] The usual cause of failure in inducing trance can be traced to misconceptions about hypnosis. Fears about the process and doubts as to its utility may instill anxiety and interfere with successful outcome. Also, if expectations about trance are not fulfilled, results may be less than optimal.

Problems amenable to hypnotic correction include habit disorders (smoking, obesity, nailbiting, insomnia, enuresis, alcoholism, teeth grinding), medical disorders (dermatologic problems, migraine, asthma and allergy, sexual dysfunction, hypertension), and psychiatric disorders (phobias, neuroses, anorexia nervosa).[26,33,34]

Hypnosis, alone or combined with chemical anesthesia, is useful in childbirth and in surgical and dental procedures. In a randomized, blind study, pain medication requirements declined in patients ". . . given instruction, suggestion and encouragement upon the severity of postoperative pain," and such patients were ready for discharge 2.7 days earlier than those not so treated.[35] In another study, pregnant women in one group were taught trance, with suggestions given for ease of delivery, comfort, and rapid healing. Another group was taught relaxation therapy alone, and a third group received only standard prenatal training. Each group contained 70 women, equalized for parity (primiparous versus multiparous). Physicians and nurses involved in the deliveries were not told to which group each woman had been assigned. Women who had been taught trance and given suggestions experienced significantly shorter first stages of labor and required significantly less pain medication than those who received prenatal training alone or relaxation instruction.[36]

Hypnosis is useful in pain control. It might be expected that the degree of pain reported when one's hand is placed in ice water, or when ischemic muscle pain is induced, should correspond to the extent of tissue damage. Sometimes it does not. In experiments in which pain was induced by those measures, McGlashan and Orne[37] and Hilgard[38,39] demonstrated that appropriate suggestions given during hypnosis can eliminate the correlation between extent of tissue damage and both the amount of reported pain and the physiologic correlates of pain.

HYPNOSIS IN PATIENTS WITH CANCER

Hypnosis has many uses in malignant disease.[26,29,33,34,40,41] It is effective against acute or chronic pain, sleeplessness, anxiety, anticipated pain or discomfort prior to surgery, radiation or chemotherapy, and feelings of helplessness and loss of control. It is not clear how pain reduction is mediated, or whether endorphins are involved. The data are contradictory; some studies show that the effects are reversed by the opiate antagonist, naloxone,[42] while others show that they are not.[43,44]

Evoking sensations previously experienced during local or spinal anesthesia can numb the affected area to pain, although usually not to touch, especially if the pain is in the same area as the previous anesthesia. The patient can be taught to experience analgesia in a glove-like distribution and to transfer the lack of sensation to the affected part. Suggestions may help the patient to "down modulate," switch off, isolate, or shrink the pain.

The duration of pain-free periods can be made to seem longer, and those of painful periods, shorter. If the pain is not serving as a "danger signal," that fact can be emphasized and the patient taught not to react to it as such. The patient will remain alert to other pains that may be danger signals which should be reported and evaluated.

The patient can learn to imagine that the painful part is "not there" (a *negative hallucination*) or "not theirs," much as a bike marathoner may do during the last few miles of a race. The patient practiced in the use of these techniques can apply them while carrying on activities of daily living. Dissociation from pain is especially useful for bedridden patients. They can re-experience other places and retrieve favorite experiences while in trance (self-induced or through the use of a tape recorded by the hypnotherapist). Often, less pain medication is required, and patients experience extended periods of alertness and comfort.

Trance techniques taught in anticipation of nausea or discomfort can be helpful.[45] A rehearsal of a planned procedure can be conducted while the patient is in trance and suggestions made to help render the procedure as comfortable as possible. Glove analgesia can be used, for example, when an IV is being placed. Cues can be taught to facilitate the patient's entry into trance when needed: the cool feeling of the hand after an alcohol swab can serve as a cue for the patient to begin glove analgesia prior to the insertion of an IV; or patients can learn to dissociate or distract themselves during the procedure.

Through these techniques, patients regain control over situations from which much control had been lost. Patients' bodies once again respond appropriately to their direction, for example, to relax. During a procedure, patients can dissociate themselves, or the offending body part, to alter sensations or to modify the time the procedure seems to take. Patients themselves can combine the benefits of autosuggestion with those of pain medication in order to alleviate pain or decrease anxiety further. This newly gained independence and power can help even bedridden patients achieve appreciation of their own capabilities and gain a heightened sense of self-control and self-respect.

Clearly, an integrated approach is needed to manage the pain of a patient with cancer. Each of the modalities previously mentioned can be applied alone or in combination to meet individual needs. Awareness of the advantages and limitations of the various modalities can help physicians select the best combination to keep the patient as active and as comfortable as possible throughout the illness.

REFERENCES

1. Melzack, R., and Wall, P.D.: Psychophysiology of pain. *In* Pain, A Source Book for Nurses and Other Health Professionals. Edited by A.K. Jacox. Boston, Little, Brown and Co., 1977, pp. 3–25.
2. Zimmerman, M.: Neurophysiology of nociception, pain, and pain therapy. *In* Advances in Pain Research and Therapy. Vol. II. Edited by J.J. Bonica, and V. Ventafridda. New York, Raven Press, 1979, pp. 13–29.
3. Whidden, A., and Sister Mary Rebecca Fidler: Pathophysiology of pain. *In*

Pain, A Source Book for Nurses and Other Health Professionals. Edited by A.K. Jacox. Boston, Little, Brown and Co., 1977, pp. 27–56.

4. Weisenberg, M.: General and theoretical concepts of pain reactions. *In* Pain, Clinical and Experimental Perspectives. Edited by M. Weisenberg. St. Louis, C.V. Mosby Co., 1975.

5. Beecher, H.K.: Pain in men wounded in battle. Ann. Surg., *123*:96–105, 1946.

6. Beecher, H.K.: Relationship of significance of wound to the pain experienced. J.A.M.A., *161*:1609–1613, 1956.

7. Chapman, C.R.: Psychologic and behavioral aspects of cancer pain. *In* Advances in Pain Research and Therapy. Vol. II. Edited by J.J. Bonica, and V. Ventafridda. New York, Raven Press, 1979, pp. 44–56.

8. Jacox, A.K.: Sociocultural and psychological aspects of pain. *In* Pain, A Source Book for Nurses and Other Health Professionals. Edited by A.K. Jacox. Boston, Little, Brown and Co., 1977, pp. 57–87.

9. Zborowski, M.: Cultural components in responses to pain. J. Soc. Issues, *8*:16–30, 1952.

10. Bonica, J.J.: Cancer pain. *In* Pain. Edited by J.J. Bonica. New York, Raven Press, 1980, pp. 335–362.

11. Marks, R.M., and Sochar, E.J.: Undertreatment of medical inpatients with narcotic analgesics. Ann. Intern. Med., *78*:173–181, 1973.

12. Jaffe, J.H.: Drug addiction and drug abuse. *In* The Pharmacological Basis of Therapeutics. 5th Ed. Edited by L.S. Goodman, and A. Gilman. New York, Macmillan Publishing Co., 1975.

13. Twycross, R.G.: Clinical experience with diamorphine in advanced malignant disease. Int. J. Clin. Pharmacol. Biopharm., *9*:184–198, 1974.

14. Mount, B.M., Ajemian, I., and Scott, J.F.: Use of the Brompton mixture in treating the chronic pain of malignant disease. Can. Med. Assoc. J., *115*:122–124, 1976.

15. Gerbershagen, H.U.: Blocks with local anesthetics. *In* Advances in Pain Research and Therapy. Vol. II. Edited by J.J. Bonica, and V. Ventafridda. New York, Raven Press, 1979, pp. 311–335.

16. Madrid, J.L., and Bonica, J.J.: Cranial nerve blocks. Ibid., 347–355.

17. Moore, D.C.: Celiac (splanchnic) plexus block with alcohol, for cancer pain and the upper abdominal viscera. Ibid., 357–371.

18. Pagni, C.A.: General comments on ablative neurosurgical procedures. Ibid., 405–423.

19. Lipton, S.: Percutaneous cervical cordotomy. Ibid., 425–437.

20. Papo, I.: Spinal posterior rhizotomy and commissural myelotomy in the treatment of cancer pain. Ibid., 439–447.

21. Papo, I.: Open cordotomy in the treatment of cancer pain. Ibid., 449–452.

22. Bricolo, A.: Medullary tractotomy for cephalic pain of malignant disease. Ibid., 453–462.

23. Sano, K.: Stereotaxic thalamolaminotomy and posteromedial hypothalmotomy for the relief of intractable pain. Ibid., 475–485.

24. Loeser, J.D.: Dorsal column and peripheral nerve stimulation for relief of cancer pain. Ibid., 499–507.

25. Ventafridda, V., et al.: Transcutaneous nerve stimulation in cancer pain. Ibid., 509–515.

26. Kroger, W.S.: Clinical and Experimental Hypnosis. Philadelphia, J.B. Lippincott, 1963.

27. Esdaile, J.: Mesmerism in India and Its Practical Application in Surgery and Medicine. Hartford, England, Silus Andrus and Son, 1850.

28. A Syllabus on Hypnosis and a Handbook of Therapeutic Suggestions. Am. Soc. Clin. Hyp. Ed. and Res. Foundation, Des Plaines, Illinois, 1973.

29. Hilgard, E.R., and Hilgard, J.R.: Hypnosis in the Relief of Pain. Los Altos, California, W.K. Kaufman, 1975.
30. Spiegel, H., and Spiegel, D.: Trance and Treatment. New York, Basic Books, 1978.
31. Shor, R.E., and Orne, E.C.: The Harvard Group Scale of Hypnotic Susceptibility, Form A. Palo Alto, California, Consulting Psychologists Press, 1962.
32. Thompson, K.: Personal communication.
33. Kroger, W.S., and Fezler, W.D.: Hypnosis and Behavior Modification: Imagery Conditioning. Philadelphia, J.B. Lippincott, 1976.
34. Hartland, J.: Medical and Dental Hypnosis and Its Clinical Applications. 2nd Ed. London, Balliere Tindall, 1971.
35. Egbert, L.D., Battit, G.E., Welch, C.E., and Bartlett, M.K.: Reduction of postoperative pain by encouragement and instruction of patients. N. Engl. J. Med., 270:825–827, 1964.
36. Williamson, J.A.: Hypnosis in Obstetrics. Nurs. Times, 71:1895–1897, 1975.
37. McGlashan, T.H., Evans, F.J., and Orne, M.T.: The nature of hypnotic analgesia and placebo response to experimental pain. Psychosom. Med., 31:227–246, 1969.
38. Hilgard, E.R.: Pain as a puzzle for psychology and physiology. Am. Psychol., 24:103–113, 1969.
39. Hilgard, E.R., and Morgan, A.H.: Heart rate and blood pressure in the study of laboratory pain in man under normal conditions as influenced by hypnosis. Acta Neurobiol. Exp., 35:741–759, 1975.
40. Crasilnick, H.B., and Hall, J.A.: Clinical Hypnosis. New York, Grune and Stratton, 1975.
41. Erickson, M.H.: An introduction to the study and application of hypnosis for pain control. *In* Hypnosis and Psychosomatic Medicine. Edited by J. Lassner. Berlin, Springer-Verlag, 1967.
42. Stephenson, J.B.P.: Reversal of hypnosis-induced analgesia by naloxone. Lancet, 2:991–992, 1978.
43. Goldstein, A., and Hilgard, E.R.: Failure of the opiate antagonist naloxone to modify hypnotic analgesia. Proc. Natl. Acad. Sci. USA, 72:2041–2043, 1975.
44. Bowsher, D.: Ability to lie on bed of nails not due to endogenous opioids. Lancet, 1:1132, 1980.
45. Ban, T., et al.: Comparison of prochlorperazine (CP) and hypnosis (H) as antiemetic therapy. Proc. Am. Soc. Clin. Onc., 22:424, 1981.

Chapter 7

Endorphins: Pharmacologic and Physiologic Implications for Pain Control

Gerard A. Ruch

The discovery of endorphins, a group of morphine-like substances produced by the body, has exciting implications for improved understanding and control of the pain experienced by many terminal cancer patients.

The presence of specific receptors for opiates in the brain was suspected nearly a decade ago when it was seen how rapidly a narcotic antagonist, such as naloxone, could bring addicts out of morphine or heroin comas. Intravenous administration of the antagonist promptly restored consciousness, improved respiration, and brought on withdrawal. Naloxone was presumed to bind to an opiate receptor site and thereby to displace the narcotic agonist. Using radioactively labelled naloxone, Pert and Snyder showed that the brain tissue of all vertebrates, but not invertebrates, had high binding affinity (receptors) for this foreign drug.[1] Surprisingly, the primitive hagfish, the oldest known vertebrate traceable at least to the Devonian period over 350 million years ago, proved to possess as much opiate-receptor binding as monkey or man.

DISCOVERY OF ENDOGENOUS OPIATES AND OPIATE RECEPTORS

The discovery of endogenous opiates followed quickly, as Hughes et al. isolated from pig brain two morphine-like agonists whose effects were blocked by naloxone.[2] They named these two pentapeptides, which differed only in their carboxyl terminal amino acid, enkephalins, from the Greek word meaning "in the head."

> Methionine enkephalin: H—Tyr—Gly—Gly—Phe—Met—OH
> Leucine enkephalin: H—Tyr—Gly—Gly—Phe—Leu—OH

Next the amino acid sequence of met-enkephalin was recognized in a polypeptide called Beta-lipotropin, isolated from pituitary glands by Li in the early 1960s. Testing of Beta-lipotropin revealed, however, that it was devoid of opiate activity, but that a fragment encompassing amino acids 61–91 was active. This fragment contained met-enkephalin (amino acids 61–65) within its sequence. Guillemin and colleagues examined extracts of pituitary and hypothalamic tissue and found that they contained a number of polypeptides with opiate activity.[3] They identified these component peptides of Beta-lipotropin as the following:

	amino acid sequence
α-endorphin:	61–76
β-endorphin:	61–91
γ-endorphin:	61–77

Currently, most researchers refer to endogenous opioids of both the enkephalin and the other types as endorphins (endogenous morphine). The structure of Beta-lipotropin is shown in Figure 7–1.

The localization of endogenous opiates in the central nervous system (CNS) was achieved by the use of antibodies and immunocytochemical mapping techniques. Barchas and others have shown that the endogenous opiates of the pituitary and brain are synthesized independently,[4] with enkephalins present in highest concentration in the brain and spinal cord, and Beta-endorphin predominating in the pituitary.

Enkephalin pathways are multiple cell groups throughout the spinal cord and brainstem connected by relatively short axons. Leu- and met-enkephalin have virtually identical distributions and

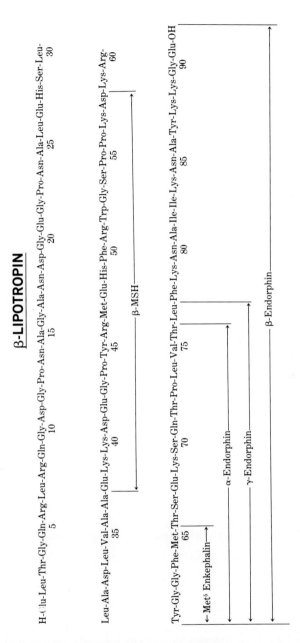

Fig. 7–1. Structures of Beta-lipotropin, endorphins, and methionine-enkephalin. (From Morley, J.E.: The endocrinology of the opiates and opioid peptides. Metabolism, *30*:195–209, 1981.)

may even be in the same neurons. The highest concentrations are found in the globus pallidus; other areas rich in enkephalins include the nucleus accumbens, the amygdala, and the medial hypothalamus. The distribution of enkephalins correlates closely with opiate receptor distribution as revealed by autoradiography. Because the enkephalins are found in brain areas involved in pain transmission, respiration, endocrine control, and mood, their role in all these activities is being actively explored. The relative instability of the enkephalins suggests that they might function as inhibitory neurotransmitters that mediate the integration of sensory information related to pain and emotional behavior.

Beta-endorphin pathways are single cell groups in the hypothalamus with long axons innervating midbrain and limbic structures.[4] The highest concentrations are found in the medial hypothalamus, with lesser amounts in the periaqueductal gray matter and locus ceruleus. Beta-endorphin is thought to be a neuromodulator; in other words, it alters neuronal activity perhaps by affecting neurotransmitter synthesis, release, receptor interactions, re-uptake, or metabolism. In addition, unlike the enkephalins which are rapidly inactivated by peptidase enzymes, endorphins are stable compounds in vivo.

TYPES OF OPIATE RECEPTORS

In 1976, Martin and colleagues postulated, on the basis of behavioral and neurophysiologic data from chronic spinal dogs, that there are at least three different opiate receptors.[6] A fourth type, delta, was described by Lord et al.[7] and by Frenk et al.[8] in the mouse vas deferens and rat brain. These receptors differ in their affinities for exogenous opiates (morphine, etc.) and endogenous opiates (peptides). Naloxone, the purest opiate receptor antagonist available, has a high affinity only for mu-type receptors. It is a somewhat weaker antagonist at kappa- and sigma-type receptors, and has virtually no effect at delta receptors. Because naloxone is a relatively "clean" drug that displays few pharmacologic actions other than opiate receptor blockade, many researchers have interpreted their results solely in light of this well-known action. However, naloxone also blocks synaptic receptors for the inhibitory neurotransmitter GABA (gamma-aminobutyrate), which probably explains the convulsant effects of high doses of this antagonist.

The different types of opiate receptors and their effects are out-lined in Table 7–1.

Opiate receptors in the CNS are found in highest density in the limbic system, specifically in the frontal and temporal cortex, amygdala, and hippocampus. Significant levels also are found in the thalamus, striatum, hypothalamus, midbrain, and spinal cord.[10] Because opiate receptors throughout the brain vary in drug spec-ificity, drugs that act selectively on individual receptor populations may provide selective therapeutic advantages in the future.

Opiate receptors also are found in the peripheral nervous sys-tem. Those in the guinea pig ileum and mouse vas deferens have been particularly well studied.

The affinity of opiates for receptors in vitro relates to the concentration of sodium ions. Initial binding experiments in brain and other tissues showed that antagonists and their corresponding agonists appeared to have the same affinity for the receptor. It was well known, however, that in vivo antagonists were much more potent than agonists. Snyder and associates resolved this paradox when they modified their technique for measuring the receptor.[11] They had conducted their initial experiments without any of the ions found abundantly in the body. As soon as they incorporated sodium ions, dramatic changes in the behavior of agonists and antagonists occurred. Thus, 100 mM sodium enhanced the binding of opiate antagonists and greatly diminished the bind-ing of agonists. These effects were selective for sodium ions (Na^+), could be mimicked somewhat by lithium ions with their similar atomic radius, but could not be mimicked by potassium, rubidium, or cesium ions.

A sodium index was developed that accurately predicts the extent to which a drug is an opiate agonist or antagonist (Fig. 7–2). The index measures the degree to which the drug inhibits binding of radioactively labelled naloxone to brain cell membrane prepa-rations in the presence and in the absence of sodium ions. A sodium index of 2, for example, means that a drug's ability to bind to the opiate receptor is reduced by half in the presence of Na^+.

Using the sodium ion index avoids the much more expensive monkey and human screening and thus greatly simplifies the search for new analgesics. It is believed that an analgesic without ad-dictive properties would be a mixed agonist/antagonist with a so-dium index of 2–5. However, two such drugs (pentazocine and ketocyclazocine) that meet these criteria may produce addiction in man.

TABLE 7-1. Types and Activity of Opiate Receptors.[8,9]

CNS opiate receptor type:	Mu	Kappa	Sigma	Delta
Agonists:	Morphine	Morphine Ketocyclazocine	N-allylnorcyclazocine (SKF 10,047)	Leu-enkephalin Met-enkephalin
Overall CNS effects:	Supraspinal analgesia; physical dependence; euphoria	Spinal analgesia Sedation	Hallucinations Delirium	Epileptic seizures
Other effects:	Decreased pulse, respiration	No pulse or respiration changes	Increased pulse, respiration	?

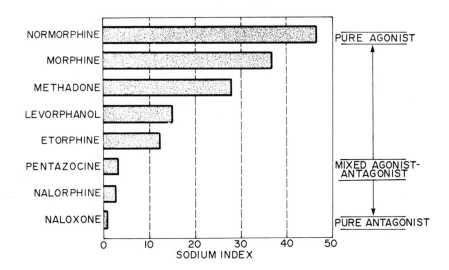

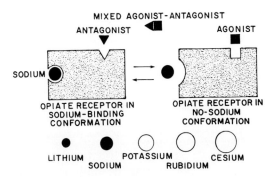

Fig. 7–2. Sodium index and model of opiate receptor. (Adapted from Snyder, S.H.: Opiate receptors and internal opiates. Sci. Am., 236:44–56, March, 1977.)

Snyder and associates have proposed that sodium acts as an allosteric effector, favoring the binding of antagonists and decreasing the binding of agonists.[10] Because the fluid bathing the cellular membranes of the brain is rich in sodium ions (Na^+), the opiate receptor is assumed to exist normally in the Na^+-binding (antagonist) state. Typical morphine effects such as analgesia and euphoria would be observed only if drugs bind to the agonist state of the receptor. By binding to the receptor in the Na^+-binding state, antagonists would reduce the number of receptors that are capable of mediating morphine effects.

The linkages between opiate receptors and physiologic responses are of intense current interest. Some opiate receptors are linked to Na^+ gating; here agonists (morphine, enkephalins, endorphins) reduce Na^+ flux across membranes (i.e., are inhibitory), whereas antagonists (naloxone, naltrexone) increase Na^+ flux (i.e., are stimulatory).[13] Opiate receptors have been described as oscillating rapidly between two distinct conformations that block or admit sodium ions, depending upon whether they are occupied by an agonist or antagonist opiate.[14] Other opiate receptors appear to be linked to adenylate cyclase;[15] here opioid agonists as well as opioid-like peptides mediate a lowering of cyclic AMP levels within neuronal cells in culture, and antagonists oppose this. Thus, cyclic AMP may be a "second messenger" for enkephalins and endorphins, as well as for many other agonists. Other unknown linkages probably exist as well.

ENDOGENOUS OPIATES AND PAIN

Morphine and other narcotic analgesics act primarily within the CNS where they block certain inhibitory pathways. These drugs are effective against pain of high intensity ("sharp pain") due to muscular spasm or distension of hollow viscera, or pain involving nerve trunks. By contrast, aspirin and similar analgesics are believed to have their primary actions outside the CNS, although a central component may be present. These drugs are effective against pain of low to moderate intensity ("dull pain"), but not against high intensity pain. The pain that aspirin-like drugs can block is usually associated with inflammatory tissue damage or processes in which chemical mediators (prostaglandins, and possibly serotonin, bradykinin, and others) are involved.

Endogenous opiates have been tested in animals for analgesic activity, using either intravenous injections or direct applications of these peptides to certain brain areas. Although analgesia has been demonstrated for almost all endogenous opiates tested, the extent of their effects varies considerably. In general, the natural enkephalins exhibit only weak and transient analgesia (approximately 5 minutes), even when injected into the ventricular or periventricular systems of brains in various species.

However, the endorphins, particularly Beta-endorphin, produce a strong analgesic effect when administered intravenously, with a potency three to four times that of morphine and a duration of two to three hours. These differences in analgesic activity may relate in part to the enkephalins' more rapid rate of enzymatic degradation in comparison to that of the endorphins. However, since the doses of Beta-endorphin required to produce analgesia and the attendant blood levels are much higher than would occur after release from the pituitary, it is unlikely that this peptide functions physiologically in pain relief.

Snyder has proposed that enkephalins, rather than endorphins, are the peptides involved in mediating pain-related CNS functions.[12] The substantia gelatinosa area, in the dorsal gray matter in layers one and two, is the first way station in the spinal cord for integrating information about pain. Both enkephalins and opiate receptors are highly concentrated in this region. Enkephalins are contained here within small interneurons whose cell bodies, axons, and terminals are all present within the substantia gelatinosa.

Enkephalins may produce their analgesic effects by blocking the release of substance P, a putative "pain transmitter." Jessell and Iversen have shown that met-enkephalin blocks the release of substance P in isolated preparations of the trigeminal nucleus,[16] a region of the brainstem that contains the terminals of pain fibers and is especially rich in substance P neurons. This effect of met-enkephalin is prevented if naloxone is added to the system. Jessell and Iversen believe that the relationship between enkephalins and substance P may be the physiologic basis for the "pain gate" in the spinal cord postulated some years ago. They have proposed that prevention of substance P release by enkephalin may be what closes the gate, as indicated in Figure 7–3.

ENDOGENOUS OPIATES AND ACUPUNCTURE ANALGESIA

Several researchers have presented indirect evidence that acupuncture can induce the release of endogenous opiates in ani-

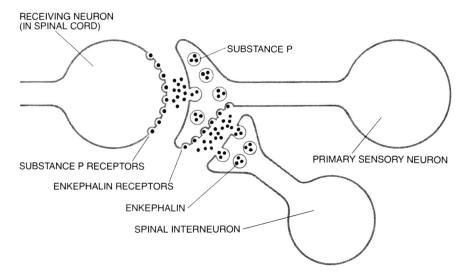

Fig. 7–3. Enkephalins may produce their analgesia by blocking the release of substance P. Furthermore, this prevention of substance P release may account for the hypothetic "pain gate" in the spinal cord. (Adapted from Iversen, L.L.: The chemistry of the brain. Sci. Am., *241*:134–149, September, 1979.)

mals and humans. Mayer et al. used electric stimulation of a tooth in human volunteers and found that acupuncture (at 2 points between thumb and index finger) could raise pain thresholds by an average of about 27%.[18] Double-blind administration of intravenous naloxone to those who had previously responded well (>20% increase in pain threshold) could antagonize the acupuncture analgesia. Because acupuncture analgesia is ineffective if the acupuncture point or peripheral nerve innervating it is rendered insensate with procaine, the authors believe that acupuncture causes the release of endogenous, centrally-acting analgesics.

Earlier, Pomerantz and Chiu had shown that analgesia can be induced in mice by electroacupuncture, suggesting the following hypothesis for acupuncture analgesia:[19] needling in appropriate points stimulates sensory nerves, which activate the pituitary or brain areas to release endogenous opiates, which reduce transmission in pain pathways.

Clement-Jones et al. obtained direct evidence indicating that acupuncture may release endorphins in the human CNS.[20] Specific radioimmunoassays were performed on lumbar cerebrospinal fluid (CSF) of ten patients with recurrent pain due to bronchial and ovarian carcinomas, estrogenic sarcoma, and other disorders. Comparison of these results with those of pain-free controls revealed no significant basal differences in Beta-endorphin or met-enkephalin levels. However, after 30 minutes of low-frequency electroacupuncture, which effectively alleviated pain, lumbar CSF Beta-endorphin levels rose significantly while the levels of met-enkephalin remained unchanged. These results suggest that analgesia produced by electroacupuncture in patients with recurrent pain may be mediated by the release of Beta-endorphin into the CSF.

ADVENT OF ENDOGENOUS OPIATE PACEMAKERS

Intractable pain in selected patients has been controlled by electric stimulation of specific brain loci. Animal experiments suggest that electric stimulation of specific periaqueductal and periventricular sites produces an analgesia comparable to that of large doses of morphine. Naloxone can partially antagonize this analgesia in most patients.[21]

Stimulation-produced analgesia (SPA) is now believed to work by releasing endogenous opioids in critical regions of the central nervous system. Akil et al. studied 30 patients with chronic pain caused by a wide range of illnesses, including low back pain, carcinoma, spinal cord injury, and arthritis.[22] Candidates were carefully screened to determine the cause of their pain, and those patients with severe psychologic problems were rejected for this treatment. Electrodes were implanted stereotaxically in a periventricular site adjacent to the posterior commissure under local anesthesia. An electrode-receiver assembly was implanted in the chest under general anesthesia. The patients were instructed in the use of a transmitter the size of a cigarette pack which is held over the embedded receiver. Eighteen of the thirty patients reported "marked" to "complete" pain relief, that is, a decrease of over 50% in their pain ratings. For many patients, 10 to 15 minutes of stimulation was as effective in relieving pain as a dose of morphine. The mean duration of analgesia was 3.8 hours, ranging from a few minutes to 24 hours. Common side effects included temperature and "tingling" paresthesias in almost half of the patients, perceived at localized sites in the face, neck, arm, or back. Most patients, however, also reported feelings of relief and relaxation, improved sleep, and increased physical activity.

In some patients, stimulation produced only transient analgesia, thus prompting them to continue the stimulation, which resulted in a loss of effectiveness within a few hours. This was avoidable in some patients by intermittent use of the stimulator at the lowest effective current level. The effect of naloxone (1 mg IV) on SPA in four subjects yielded somewhat ambiguous results. Overall, however, the antagonist appeared to lessen the analgesia. Analysis of ventricular CSF in 8 patients revealed that 20 minutes of SPA produced a significant rise in an enkephalin-like material.

Hosobuchi et al. obtained similar clinical results in patients with pain of peripheral origin (carcinoma of rectum, colon, etc.).[23] Electrodes were implanted in the periaqueductal gray matter to produce SPA. After 15 minutes of stimulation, levels of Beta-endorphin in the ventricular CSF rose 50 to 300% above baseline. No changes in enkephalin levels were detected.

Akil's[24] and earlier studies provide some evidence that the baseline levels of endogenous opioids in the CSF (and thus presumably in the brain) are depressed in patients with persistent pain. Thus, it has been speculated that endogenous opioids, either enkephalins and/or Beta-endorphin, are responsible for the analgesia obtained by patients with pain when they self-administer current to selected brain regions. However, the variable results obtained to date, as well as the variability of naloxone's effects, suggest that more than one pain system may be involved in stimulation-produced analgesia.

ENDOGENOUS OPIATES AS ANALGESICS

An early hope was that these peptides might be nonaddictive analgesics that could replace opiates in medical practice. However, animals treated with natural enkephalins or Beta-endorphin demonstrate both tolerance and dependence. Withdrawal symptoms (shaking and diarrhea) following cessation of drug administration occur after sustained exposure to these opioids.

During the last few years many enkephalin derivatives have been synthesized in an attempt to produce potent and orally active, nonaddictive analgesics. Several interesting compounds have emerged from fragment condensation methods. FK 33–824 is an orally active met-enkephalin analog developed by Sandoz.[25] It has a prolonged duration (four to five hours) of analgesic effect following IV administration to monkeys, and appears to be about twice as potent as subcutaneous morphine in the mouse and rat. In addition, it is a more potent analgesic parenterally than Beta-endorphin, and it is active even after oral administration. In self-administration testing of monkeys, however, FK 33–824 produced tolerance over a period of five weeks. Saline substitution for the drug or naloxone IV produced a marked withdrawal syndrome resembling that observed following opiate withdrawal.

Retro-inverso-enkephalinamides are a new class of potent analogs of the enkephalins, some of which are active not only subcutaneously and intravenously, but also orally. These compounds, described by Chorev et al.,[26] are internally rearranged met-enkephalin analogs in which the peptide bond between residues 4 and 5 is reversed. This partial reversal of the peptide bonds of the molecule's backbone results in enhanced activity compared to the parent compound and confers marked resistance to proteolytic degradation. Preliminary testing of certain enkephalinamides shows them to be longer acting than most enkephalin analogs studied to date. Their dependence liability is unknown.

The development of orally active enkephalins represents a major achievement in peptide chemistry. Common chemical wisdom would have argued that peptides are too readily degraded by proteolytic enzymes and too electrically charged to be absorbed from the gastrointestinal tract, escape hepatic metabolism, and penetrate into the CNS.

Another approach to increase free, and thus presumably effective, levels of enkephalins for analgesic and other clinical effects may come through the search for enkephalinase inhibitors.[27] Enkephalins may be degraded by a wide variety of nonspecific peptidases. However, several specific enkephalinases have been identified in brain membranes. Thus, a potential "analgesic of the future" might act by specifically inhibiting these enkephalinases.

ENDOGENOUS OPIATES AND THE PLACEBO RESPONSE TO PAIN

In 1978, Levine, Gordon, and Fields obtained indirect evidence suggesting that the placebo response to pain may be mediated by endogenous opioids, at least in some placebo-responsive patients.[28] They studied 51 patients who had just had wisdom teeth extracted. Treated double-blind, the patients received intravenously either morphine, a placebo (saline), or naloxone. The patients rated their own pain relief, using a ten-point scale ("no pain" to "worst pain ever"). As expected, about one third of the patients receiving the placebo reported a significant reduction in pain. All patients who had received placebos (responders and non-responders alike) were then given naloxone. The investigators found that those who had not responded to the placebo initially experienced no increase in pain with naloxone. But those individuals who were helped previously by the placebo suddenly experienced increased levels of pain. Levine et al. concluded that the observed effect in the placebo-responsive patients resulted from naloxone's ability to block the actions of endogenous opioids. Apparently, endogenous opioids had been released in response to placebo treatment. Questions remain, however. What sort of person, under what circumstances, responds best to placebos? Why can a placebo presumably trigger the release of endogenous opioids in some people and not in others? Do placebo-responders differ from non-responders in the location, quantity, types, and affinities of the specific opiate receptors involved in pain transmission?

One might also question the dosage of naloxone (10 mg) used in Levine's experiment, because less than 1 mg of the antagonist suffices to produce reversal of heroin overdosage and also block analgesia produced by opiates. It may be, however, that higher naloxone concentrations are required to compete with endogenous opioids than with exogenous opioids at receptor sites.[29]

NEW ANALGESICS

The search for new synthetic analgesics is an important by-product of recent work in opiate receptors. The discovery that low concentrations of sodium ions selectively differentiate the actions of agonists, antagonists, and mixed agonist-antagonists is being utilized in the search for less addictive opiate analgesics. Hope remains for the synthesis of a nonaddicting agonist-antagonist with a high analgesic efficacy applicable to chronic pain. Until recently, pentazocine (Talwin) was the only mixed agonist-antagonist available in the United States for clinical use. Pentazocine is believed to act as a weak competitive antagonist at the mu receptor, a strong agonist at the kappa receptor, and a weaker agonist at the sigma receptor (psychotomimetic effects).[30] Its side effects, particularly sedation, and psychotomimetic actions that produce anxiety, nightmares, and hallucinations have limited its use in some patients. Although originally believed to be free of addiction risk, clinical experience, particularly with self-administered parenteral penta-zocine, has proved otherwise.

A "second generation" of mixed agonist-antagonist opiates in-cludes butorphanol (Stadol), nalbuphine (Nubain), and buprenor-phine (Temgesic).[31,32] These drugs have a high affinity only for the mu-type receptor, but possess a low intrinsic activity there. In other words, they are partial agonists. These partial agonists can cause some antagonism to morphine by displacing it at the mu receptor, and thus are described as agonists-antagonists in this context. Although their analgesic efficacy is slightly less than that of full agonists (morphine, methadone, etc.), limited clinical ex-perience with these newer drugs suggests a lower incidence of side effects such as nausea and respiratory depression. At present, these three partial agonists appear to have a low abuse potential, less than that of codeine or propoxyphene, although reports of dependence with chronic usage have been published.

Some of the newer synthetic analgesics probably will be useful in the management of terminal cancer patients. However, many clinicians and patients may continue to prefer the euphoria and tranquility that older narcotics produce. These actions represent clinical assets that the newer drugs lack.

Clinical Benefits of Current Endorphin/Opiate Receptor Research

One of the mysteries that current research in this area may unravel concerns the development of tolerance produced by the chronic administration of opiates. Although little is known at pres-ent regarding the mechanisms of tolerance, several hypotheses have been proposed.[13] For example, the numbers and/or affinities of certain types of opiate receptors may be reduced by chronic administration of these agonists. Alternatively, an uncoupling of the binding to the receptor and its normally-linked physiologic responses may occur.

Derivatives of endogenous opioids themselves, manipulation of their levels by pharmacologic or other means, or the synthesis of selective opiate receptor agonists-antagonists may well provide more effective and specific pain control in the future.

REFERENCES

1. Pert, C.B., and Snyder, S.H.: Opiate receptor: its demonstration in nervous tissue. Science, 179:1011–1014, 1973.
2. Hughes, J.W., et al.: Identification of two related pentapeptides from the brain with potent opiate agonist activity. Nature, 255:577–579, 1975.
3. Morley, J.E.: The endocrinology of the opiates and opioid peptides. Metabolism, 30:195–209, 1981.
4. Barchas, J.D., et al.: Behavioral neurochemistry: neuroregulators and behavioral states. Science, 200:964–973, 1978.
5. Kosterlitz, H.W., and Hughes, J.: Some thoughts on enkephalin, the endogenous ligand. Life Sci., 17:91–96, 1975.
6. Martin, W.R., et al.: The effects of morphine- and nalorphine-like drugs in the non-dependent and morphine-dependent chronic spinal dog. J. Pharmacol. Exp. Ther., 197:517–532, 1976.
7. Lord, J.A.H.: Endogenous opioid peptides: multiple agonists and receptors. Nature, 267:495–499, 1977.
8. Frenk, H., McCarty, B.L., and Liebeskind, J.C.: Different brain areas mediate the analgesic and epileptic properties of enkephalin. Science, 200:335–337, 1978.
9. Jaffe, J.H., and Martin, W.R.: Opioid analgesics and antagonists. In The Pharmacological Basis of Therapeutics. Edited by A.G. Gilman, L.S. Goodman, and A. Gilman. New York, MacMillan, 1980.
10. Snyder, S.H., et al.: The opiate receptor. Ann. Intern. Med., 81:534–540, 1974.
11. Snyder, S.H.: The opiate receptor and morphine-like peptides in the brain. Am. J. Psychiatry, 135:645–652, 1978.
12. Snyder, S.H.: Opiate receptors and internal opiates. Sci. Am., 236:44–56, March, 1977.
13. Spector, S.: Opiate receptors and their clinical implications. Circ. Res., 46:I-138–141, (Supp. I) 1980.
14. Bunney, W.E.: Basic and clinical studies of endorphins. Ann. Intern. Med., 91:239–250, 1979.
15. Sharma, S.K., et al.: Dual regulation of adenylate cyclase accounts for narcotic dependence and tolerance. Proc. Natl. Acad. Sci. USA, 72:3092–3096, 1975.
16. Jessell, T.M., and Iversen, L.L.: Opiate analgesics inhibit substance P release from rat trigeminal nucleus. Nature, 268:549–551, 1977.
17. Iversen, L.L.: The chemistry of the brain. Sci. Am., 241:134–149, September, 1979.
18. Mayer, D.J., et al.: Antagonism of acupuncture analgesia in man by the narcotic antagonist naloxone. Brain Res., 121:368–372, 1977.
19. Pomeranz, B., and Chiu, D.: Naloxone blockade of acupuncture analgesia: endorphin implicated. Life Sci., 19:1757–1762, 1976.
20. Clement-Jones, V., et al.: Increased Beta-endorphin but not Met-enkephalin levels in human cerebrospinal fluid after acupuncture for recurrent pain. Lancet, 2:946–948, 1980.
21. Mayer, D.J., et al.: Analgesia from electrical stimulation in the brainstem of the rat. Science, 174:1351–1354, 1971.
22. Akil, H., Richardson, D.E., and Barchas, J.D.: Pain control by focal brain stimulation in man: relationship to enkephalins and endorphins. In Mechanisms of Pain and Analgesic Compounds. Edited by R.F. Beers, Jr., and E.G. Bassett. New York, Raven Press, 1979.
23. Hosobuchi, Y., et al.: Stimulation of human periaqueductal gray for pain

relief increases immunoreactive Beta-endorphin in ventricular fluid. Science, *203*:279–281, 1979.

24. Akil, H., et al.: Enkephalin-like material in ventricular cerebrospinal fluid of pain patients after analgetic focal stimulation. Science, *201*:463–465, 1978.
25. Roemer, D., et al.: A synthetic enkephalin analogue with prolonged parenteral and oral analgesic activity. Nature, *268*:547–549, 1977.
26. Chorev, M., et al.: Partially modified retro-inverso enkephalinamides: topochemical long-acting analogs *in vitro* and *in vivo*. Science, *204*:1210–1212, 1979.
27. Snyder, S.H.: Clinical relevance of opioid receptor and opioid peptide research. Nature, *279*:13–14, 1979.
28. Levine, J.D., Gordon, N.C., and Fields, H.L.: The mechanism of placebo analgesia. Lancet, *2*:654–657, 1978.
29. Goldstein, A.: Endorphins and pain: a critical review. *In* Mechanisms of Pain and Analgesic Compounds. Edited by R.F. Beers, Jr., and E.G. Bassett. New York, Raven Press, 1979.
30. Martin, W.R.: History and development of mixed opioid agonists, partial agonists and antagonists. Br. J. Clin. Pharmacol., *7*:273S–279S, 1979.
31. Lewis, J.R.: Evaluation of new analgesics. Butorphanol and nalbuphine. J.A.M.A., *243*:1465–1467, 1980.
32. Jasinski, D.R.: Human pharmacology and abuse potential of the analgesic buprenorphine. Arch. Gen. Psychiatry, *35*:501–516, 1978.

Chapter 8

Psychosocial Problems

Barrie R. Cassileth
James L. Stinnett

The current discontent with the American health care system,[1] and probably the growing involvement of many patients with unorthodox therapies as well, stems in part from increased technologic advance resulting in highly specialized professional functions. This has led to narrowly defined clinical roles and to a longing common among patients for the less clinically sophisticated, but more personally satisfying, kind of doctor-patient relationship typical of past decades.

In many respects, "psychosocial support" is a modern euphemism for the qualities of human warmth, caring, and interpersonal skills characteristic of the bygone doctor-patient interaction. At no time is the patient's need for this kind of support more pressing than during terminal illness. Ironically, at no point throughout the span of illness and treatment is that support less available from primary caregivers than during the terminal phase. Other professionals are available to deal with the dying patient's psychologic needs—psychiatrists, social workers, clergy, even thanatologists—and the temptation is great to call upon them, in order to justify our decreasing contact as the patient slips clinically beyond capacity for therapeutic intervention.

The sense that true professionalism excludes emotional involvement, the perception that time and skills are more efficiently and effectively spent with aggressively-treatable patients, and the absence of training and guidelines for helpful interactions with dying patients leave us unarmed, unschooled, and uncomfortable.

A large body of data exists, much of it based on solid studies of terminally ill patients, that provides helpful information on the needs of such patients and on how clinicians can interact most beneficially.

This chapter is approached from a perspective involving three general premises. First, that the business of *living*, of sustaining or enriching relationships and of maximizing remaining time, is the proper focus of energies and goals for the terminal patient and the clinician. Second, that dying is not a psychiatric disorder, and labels of psychologic dysfunction have little place or utility in the care of the terminally ill. Third, that the clinician's responsibility for the terminal patient includes psychosocial support, and such support is a legitimate and feasible portion of the physician's obligation.

A caveat is in order, however, with regard to the final premise. Although every patient requires and deserves the physician's continued support, not every patient requires special or additional intervention. Many people have the inner resources and family support not only to manage well on their own, but even to help others in the process. Many patients exhibit striking and surprising degrees of psychic strength and resourcefulness.

With today's emphasis on death and the current popularity of publications on the subject, the danger exists that an individual's behavior may be judged deficient or incorrect against some theoretic norm of what is "appropriate" or "healthy" during the final phase of life. The possibility of this danger is increased by overzealous interpretation of Elisabeth Kubler-Ross's analysis of the stages of death.[2] This pioneering work, despite the author's explicit warning, is readily perverted into the simplistic notion that people go neatly from one stage to another, and that anyone out of step requires psychologic assistance. Not all patients experience particular stages of emotional response, and some remain comfortably fixed in a single emotional niche. The individual's own comfort, judged against a highly personalized standard, must guide assessment. Whether an individual conforms to a general or idealized prototype of the "dying patient," if indeed one exists, is neither relevant nor helpful.

COMMUNICATION

The area of communication exemplifies two extremes of a problem highlighted by the contemporary focus on death and dying.

On the one hand, there is a tendency to expect and encourage all patients to verbalize their concerns and feelings about death; on the other hand, there is a preference among the more traditionally schooled to avoid any such discussion at all costs. Neither approach, indiscriminately applied, can serve the best interests of patients.

The nonverbal individual—the person whose feelings throughout life have remained matters of the utmost privacy or the intellectual who finds comfort in removing personal experience to a universal or literary plane—is inappropriately pressed to discuss how *"you* feel about *your* impending death."[3] The other extreme tendency is perhaps more common: our frequent inability or unwillingness to admit to the patient that we know he is dying.

This may be the new conspiracy of silence. The issue is no longer whether to reveal a cancer diagnosis, but rather how to acknowledge to patients the sorrow and importance of their impending death. This is an aspect of communication difficult not only for clinicians, but for patients' friends and relatives as well. Forced to deal alone with the magnitude of their situation and with its terrible sadness, such patients are truly abandoned even in the midst of good clinical care and attentive family and staff. The conspiracy of silence denies patients the opportunity to ventilate and share concerns if they wish to do so. It cuts them off not only from meaningful communication with others, but also from the relief that the act of sharing one's concerns and feelings typically brings. This unwillingness or inability to talk about death, or to allow patients to do so, contributes to the fear of abandonment that, along with fears of pain, represents dying patients' most prevalent concern.

Many find the subject of death uncomfortable because it is difficult to know what to say. We dread the "why me?" questions that patients may ask, and we ourselves may harbor the same "why this patient?" doubts. As clinicians, we are accustomed to ready answers, and here there are none at all. What dying patients need and want from us, however, is not answers but concern and interest. The challenge is less what to say than how to listen.

There are some specific points of explanation and reassurance that many patients welcome. Patients need to be assured of their physician's continuing involvement and participation in their care. The dying patient, moved to a room at the end of the hospital corridor and visited by staff with decreasing frequency and for ever shorter periods of time, is by now a time-worn story, but it remains a persistent reality in many instances.

Explicit assurance that pain will be continuously monitored and controlled, accompanied of course by action toward that promise, is profoundly relieving to patients who recall the long-standing agonies of a dying relative years ago, or whose primary association with terminal cancer is lingering, painful death. Few patients ask directly, but many worry privately, about the specifics of how they will die. One patient with leukemia, then at home, feared for months that his death would occur suddenly, possibly while driving his wife and children in their car, and that he would destroy his entire family as a result of his own sudden death. He was greatly relieved to learn that death would occur gradually, and that adequate time would be available to prepare and protect his family.

Patients and families are reassured also to learn that death is almost invariably preceded by gradual loss of function and by peace and tranquility. It is devoid of fear or anguish, an observation made by Osler and many others.[4,5] Many fear suffocation, which is a realistic concern about a problem that can be managed (see Chapters 2 and 17). Other patients have expressed the irrational fear that, while receiving palliative radiation therapy, the radiation apparatus might fall on them or that no one would know if they were in distress and in need of help.

Patients often harbor frightening fantasies, such as that of sudden death, which are readily correctable. Fantasies and similar concerns can be handled, but only if we know what they are. Such knowledge requires giving patients the opportunity to talk and to voice their worries, which in turn requires our willingness to be there and listen.

ALIENATION AND LOSS OF CONTROL

The almost total dependency of the hospitalized terminally ill patient causes frustration and humiliation, particularly for those whose lives have been characterized by independence and decision-making for self and others. Hospitalization even for short-term, minor ailments is associated with anxiety, alienation, loss of control, and the disquiet induced by unintelligible terminology used in reference to oneself.

All of these problems are exacerbated for terminally ill patients who face also a childlike existence in which physical needs are attended to by others; in which relief from pain and discomfort depends upon people and actions outside of themselves; and in which progressive debilitation increasingly narrows their sphere of independent capacity and action. Appeals for "death with dignity" and "quality of remaining life," as well as the popularity of hospice, in part are attributable to these facts of terminal hospitalization.

The sense of alienation and loss of control can be decreased at least to a degree, but usually at some cost to the efficiency of hospital routine. Patients should be given the opportunity to make decisions whenever possible. For example, in the absence of therapeutic preference, the patient should have the option to receive medication in liquid versus capsule form. Patients should be given the opportunity to medicate themselves when feasible, and should have copies of their own medication schedules. Whenever possible, self-care and the opportunity to select preferred menus also help the patient regain some control over the environment and the disease. Removing from a patient all opportunity to act independently defeats the goal of enabling patients to maximize their remaining time and to "live" until they die. The patient who is rendered totally dependent to suit institutional needs is socially "dead" before his time.

TYPES OF DEATH

Pattison delineates four definitions of death,[6] a conceptualization that is clinically useful as well as theoretically interesting. The first, "sociologic death," constitutes the withdrawal and separation from the patient by others. Depending on the patient's physical environment and the reactions of family and staff, sociologic death can last for days or weeks if the patient is left alone to die; for years if the patient has been abandoned, unvisited, in a nursing home; or for minutes if the patient remains surrounded by caring others until the moment of death.

Second, there is "psychic death," in which patients accept death as imminent and regress into themselves. Usually psychic and actual death occur almost simultaneously, but some patients give up, accept death prematurely, and refuse to continue living. "Biologic death," the third type, is defined as the absence of cognitive function or awareness, although artificial support systems may sustain vital organ functioning. Fourth is "physiologic death," wherein all vital organs have ceased to function.

The ordinary sequence of events proceeds from sociologic

through physiologic death, but distortions of this process can occur. Inappropriately early sociologic death, for example, is a common phenomenon as just described, or when family members, given a projected length of survival, find the patient still alive months after the expected time limit has elapsed (see Chapter 10). This problem can be precluded by avoiding specific projections of survival time such as, "He has approximately four months to live." Psychic death can occur prematurely for patients who view a cancer diagnosis as stigmatizing and tantamount to immediate demise. If recognized, such emotional reactions are reversible.

GUILT

Adults as well as children may interpret terminal illness, particularly terminal malignant disease, as punishment for past failures or actions. The impact of this kind of thinking has been magnified in recent years by popularization of the notion that maintaining and regaining health are primarily the individual's responsibilities. Although we are responsible for behaviors that carry health risks, such as smoking, diet, and lack of exercise, the popularized notion unfortunately also embodies the precept that one is at fault personally not only for having contracted cancer, but also for failing to achieve cure.

A schoolteacher with metastatic melanoma requested a psychotherapeutic interview. She had a single, straightforward question: "Did I do this to myself by working too hard for the past ten years?" Her question received an emphatic "no." Demonstrably relieved, she was unburdened of massive guilt carried secretly since her diagnosis some months before. The guilt had been inspired by a newspaper article sponsoring the view that all illness is self-inflicted, and that cancer is incurable only if one strives inadequately or ineffectively to overcome it.

Psychosocial factors no doubt contribute in an as-yet-unknown manner to the etiology of disease, but only as one link in a long causal chain. The direct relationship postulated by some, that emotional deficit or improper lifestyle causes malignant disease, is untenable. Worse, it adds the burden of guilt to the patient already struggling with the physical and emotional difficulties of terminal illness.

ALTERNATIVE CANCER THERAPIES

The natural corollary to the notion that cancer is caused by psychosocial factors is that cancer can be cured through the patient's mental and physical efforts. This has resulted in the use of mind-control, dietary, and internal cleanliness efforts to treat cancer, which are characteristic of alternative cancer treatments today. It is interesting that current unorthodox therapies differ substantially from alternative remedies offered throughout the past century. Previous unorthodox treatments were "medicines," or at least "medicinal." They came in ampules, vials, or syringes; they were visual duplicates of standard medications, administered in the usual clinical fashion and sold by people in white coats.

Today's alternative remedies implicitly and explicitly reject any association with standard treatment. Proponents emphasize the distinction and distance of these remedies from anything medical. These are anti-medicines. The new alternative therapies involve no agents requiring FDA approval; they emphasize dietary proscription and recommendation; and they involve procedures and techniques that can be self-administered or handled by people with no particular training. These therapies, therefore, cannot be categorized as quasi- or illegitimately medical, but rather as aspects of lifestyle, beyond licensing or regulation.

It is no coincidence that the alternative cancer treatments popular today reflect an anti-medicine, pro-self-help bias. Acceptance of contemporary unorthodox approaches occurs in the context of an increasingly depersonalized and unsatisfying health care system (Chapter 13), and during a period of mounting public distrust of a medical establishment that has failed to find a cure for cancer, despite substantial time and financial support.

Alternative therapies implicitly address two important deficiencies in the traditional system, deficiencies that deeply concern cancer patients. They do so by maintaining personalized interest in patients as people, and by focusing on patients' self-involvement in or control over their disease. Patients receiving alternative treatments are required to maintain responsibility for their own care through exquisitely detailed and highly specialized dietary regimens, internal cleansing techniques, and/or mental exercises; and they receive from their alternative therapists the kind of whole-patient concern that they find missing in the traditional doctor-patient relationship.

COPING

Our ability to help patients cope demands just those qualities that patients find wanting in the traditional medical setting, and that they find more readily available from alternative therapists. The capacity to sit and listen runs contrary to our activist, interventionist orientation. The simple act of sitting down with a patient carries important meaning: it suggests a willingness and readiness for real communication. But clinicians typically stand at the bedside, and this posture itself conveys a message that is rarely misinterpreted. The patient knows that the physician is too busy with more important matters to sit down and talk. It is a unique patient who can share concerns in a meaningful and productive fashion with an individual looming over the bed, demonstrating by posture the hope and expectation of a quick departure.

Patients' needs differ from one day to the next, and each patient is unlike the other. Helpful interaction requires some understanding of the emotional status and needs of a particular patient at that point in time, understanding that can be achieved by a willingness to listen and to confront issues that are as difficult for the physician as for the patient.

The terminal patient faces a crisis of major proportions and the overwhelming prospect of extinction. It is a natural survival technique for all of us under great stress to segment the overall problem or task, and to deal with smaller, more manageable pieces of the whole on a sequential basis. Our approach to terminal patients can help them similarly to deal with manageable segments of the whole. We can guide them through incremental disappointments, each of which can be mastered before the next problem is confronted. Patients can be helped to avoid the need to face one massive loss by the manner and timing of our presentation of information. Time during which to adjust to incremental loss is important and necessary. We can be guided successfully by assessing how much this patient is ready to be told at this particular point, and by knowing where the patient is in the continuum of adjustment to incremental disappointment. The goal is to obviate the patient's need to confront the totality of the loss all at once.

Patients readjust their self-perceptions and goals according to their changing clinical status. It is often difficult for the healthy outsider to understand how and where terminal patients find reason for hope or for setting goals. Patients do, however, reorient themselves and establish goals, such as going home or living to an anniversary, that are consonant with their physical realities.

Denying or minimizing the seriousness of the situation is a common and adaptive coping mechanism that also gives patients time to assimilate the impact of sequential implications of illness. Temporary denial affords the opportunity to marshal psychologic resources needed to deal with the problem. Temporary denial among seriously ill patients is not psychopathologic; it serves a useful and adaptive purpose by buffering the impact of new realities. Denial gives patients time to cope with small setbacks, postponing the need to face the entire problem at one time, and should not be interfered with. House staff occasionally are alarmed by patients who they conclude are doing poorly because they "won't talk about their dying." Not all patients talk about "their dying" when one might think they should, and some patients never verbalize the subject. If the mechanism of denial makes the patient more comfortable and does not interfere with care, it should be respected and left alone. The well-meaning bias to help the patient "confront reality" should not be used as a rationale to batter successful adaptive defenses.

Anger is a natural response to massive disappointment and impending loss. Because it is difficult for rational people to display anger at something as inexplicable and abstract as fate or terminal disease, anger tends to be displaced onto potentially more controllable concrete or neutral aspects of the patient's environment, such as caregivers, hospital food or routine, or family members. We need to respond to patient's anger, but to its real rather than superficial meaning. Assaults should not be taken personally, nor dealt with at face value. Instead of reacting to the patient's words, for example by apologizing for inadequately hot food, we should respond by confronting the source of the anger ("I know you're angry. It's awful to be so sick, and I feel terrible about it too.") Anger is another coping response that helps the patient gain mastery and control over an essentially uncontrollable situation.

Another type of effort to attain mastery is the attempt to find purpose or meaning in the illness and impending death. The meaning may be perceived in terms of religious faith or some other, highly personal, construct. If the ascribed meaning is detrimental, for example if it involves guilt or self-blame for the disease, efforts on the part of the clinician and possibly outside intervention are needed to reorient the patient to a more reasonable and comfortable perspective. Typically, however, patients find purpose or meaning in their suffering in such a way as to provide spiritual or emotional relief, and they should be supported toward this goal.

Important individual differences color patients' needs and reactions. Cultural and situational factors modify pain thresholds, pain perception, and need for analgesics (Chapter 6). The symbolic implications of cancer influence the meaning ascribed to the disease, readiness to comply with therapeutic regimens, and general emotional response.[7] Family support and demands, personality, lifestyle and internal resources, and habitual modes of coping with crisis help determine the quality of adaptation, the effectiveness of coping, the need for intervention, and the type of preferred doctor-patient relationship. Patients vary in their preferences for detailed information and in the extent to which they want to participate in treatment decisions.[8]

The needs and strengths of terminally ill patients are diverse. As such, each patient must be approached not according to some predetermined notion of "correct" attitudes and behavior, but through sensitivity to the unique qualities of the particular individual. In addition, just as different patients vary, an individual patient's needs and emotional status will change substantially over time. Fluctuations are to be expected. A standard or uniform approach to patients, or even to a single patient across time, is no more appropriate than an invariant style of communication with one's colleagues or family.

Understanding what the patient is experiencing and serving that patient well demand professional role flexibility, emotional accessibility, the capacity to listen, and a readiness to share and thereby help diminish grief. These are skills that we tend to have as individuals, but skills that are foreign to medical training and to our usual sense of what physicians should do and be. The physician must remain with the patient, continue to participate in management, and sustain contact throughout the terminal phase so that the patient's fear of abandonment is not realized.

The patient's death is not our failure nor that of the medical system. The guilt we may feel when impending death gnaws as a personal or professional failure is misplaced. Patients want and require of their physicians continued concern and attention. Patients assign blame and disappointment not to our inability to repel inevitable death, but to our discomfort and reluctance to share with them its tribulations and grief.

REFERENCES

1. Knowles, J.H.: Doing Better and Feeling Worse: Health in the United States. Daedalus, Winter, 1977 (entire volume).
2. Kubler-Ross, E.: On Death and Dying. New York, Macmillan Publishing Co., 1969.
3. Hudson, R.P.: Death, dying, and the zealous phase. Ann. Intern. Med., 88:696–702, 1978.
4. Thomas, L.: Notes of a biology watcher: the long habit. N. Engl. J. Med., 286:825–826, 1972.
5. Parkes, C.M.: Psychological aspects. In Psychosocial Care of the Dying Patient. Edited by C.A. Garfield. New York, McGraw-Hill, 1978.
6. Pattison, E.M. The living-dying process. In Psychosocial Care of the Dying Patient. Edited by C.A. Garfield. New York, McGraw-Hill, 1978.
7. Cassileth, B.R.: The evolution of oncology as a sociomedical phenomenon. In The Cancer Patient: Social and Medical Aspects of Care. Edited by B.R. Cassileth. Philadelphia, Lea & Febiger, 1979.
8. Cassileth, B.R., Zupkis, R.V., Sutton-Smith, K., and March, V.: Information and participation preferences among cancer patients. Ann. Intern. Med., 92:832–836, 1980.

Chapter 9

The Role of the Family Therapist

Tovia G. Freedman

Serious illness impacts critically not only on the patient, but also on all members of the patient's family and on the family system as a whole. Starting as a crisis at the time of diagnosis, the family's problem, like the disease itself, can become chronic, encompassing, and debilitating. The family therapist can play a unique role with the family confronting a terminal illness. As a non-medical professional, the family therapist can join the family system to assist with the many changes and transitions that the family system will experience from diagnosis to the patient's death and throughout the bereavement period. Maintaining a non-pathologic view of the family system, the family therapist focuses on developing existing strengths, rather than on the family's weaknesses or inadequacies. In the face of dysfunctional response, the therapist strives to assist the family toward helpful change.

Family systems theory enables a view of the patient not as an isolated individual, but as an interacting and reacting member of a mutually-dependent unit. This conceptual framework enhances understanding of the role that illness plays in the family and helps clarify the need for and direction of necessary interventions. Applying a systems model, the family therapist views the individual patient in the context of the family system. This approach is analogous to treating a particular clinical problem after assessing the patient's total physiologic status and needs.

The term "family" contains present and historic connotations, as well as conscious and unconscious meaning. The family may be defined as a system or group of individuals who are bound to one another emotionally and functionally. This includes friends and others who play significant roles. Encompassed also are those silent members whom the patient or others may describe as disinterested or unavailable, such as those who fail to call and are important by virtue of their absence. The impact on the family system of these silent or invisible others cannot be ignored.

Every family develops a unique style and structure based on its values, history, and beliefs. This structure is seen in the patterns of interaction among members of the system. The structure of the family system is revealed in verbal and nonverbal communication patterns, as well as in intra-family power relationships, alliances, and subsystems. These characteristics are most apparent in the roles assumed by individual family members and in interactions among family members. The family will continue to function so long as established roles continue to be fulfilled and members continue to interact in accordance with that family's rules for the system. This necessitates flexibility on the part of family members so that roles become interchangeable.

TERMINAL ILLNESS: A FAMILY EVENT

Family history, style, and previous experiences with illness contribute to the family's ability to handle terminal illness. Family adaptation to terminal illness is functional or dysfunctional depending on how the disease is incorporated into the family's structure and on what role the illness plays in maintaining the family system. The functional family, even though it may experience periods of stress that cause disorder, manages overall to incorporate the disease into its lifestyle, not allowing it to control the family. It manages also to adapt to consequent changes in the sick individual, in other family members, and therefore in the entire family system. The dysfunctional family, although it may experience periods of adaptation, displays inability on both an individual and a family basis to continue with life's tasks. Thus, dysfunction reflects rigidity in the "rules" by which the family operates, rigidity that is significant enough to interfere with the family's ability to adjust to change.[1]

A family's response to terminal illness is congruent with that family's pattern of reaction to other crisis situations, and the degree of dysfunctional response to terminal illness can be anticipated on the basis of previous reactions to other unexpected, undesirable events. Serious illness superimposes strains which often bring covert, unresolved problems to light, and which magnify existing flaws or weaknesses in family structure. In some instances, however, serious illness may serve as an impetus to strengthen family structure and ties.

Knowledge of the family's previous style of adaptation to crisis and of its capacity for flexibility assists assessment of the patient's and family's needs. It is within the family that both growth and healing occur.[2] The family system and its subsystems strive naturally toward homeostasis.[3] A functional family is able to incorporate stress by adapting to transitional phases of imbalance, and by moving toward a new homeostasis. All families experience various periods of function and dysfunction, which relate to the developmental stages that a family goes through over time and to its ability to incorporate change. In families that tend to be rigid rather than flexible, terminal illness may deter return to homeostasis and may induce serious and prolonged dysfunction.

Because every family is unique, the reaction to and the effect of the diagnosis vary. The implication of the diagnosis is tantamount to an assault on the roots of the family system. The family must not only survive this initial, acute crisis; it must also incorporate the long-term burden of illness over time. Impending death due to chronic illness, as opposed to sudden death by heart attack or accident, permits a period of time during which changes in the family system and gradual adjustment may occur.

Hopefully, the family will begin to move toward homeostasis as a routine of care is established for the patient. However, changes in the patient's condition and consequent adjustments in medical treatment may unbalance the family anew. This "roller coaster" syndrome is emotionally fatiguing for the family and makes homeostasis difficult to maintain.

Knowledge of the family's needs and interpersonal dependencies is critical in assisting the family to regain homeostasis and in determining need for intervention. What support systems exist?[4] What is each family member's relationship with the patient? What supports and conflicts exist in these relationships? How does each family member conceptualize the patient's impending death? How will family roles change during the final stage of illness and after the patient's death? How has the family resolved conflict in the past? How do family members deal with anger, aggression, and hostility?

All of the emotional and concrete resources that a patient and family can gather are taxed during a terminal illness. The patient's fears and anxieties may result in excessive regression, dependence, projection, denial, and magical expectations. Many psychologic symptoms seen in the patient, such as regression and denial, are displayed by family members as well. The patient's spouse, children, or parents may revert to dysfunctional behaviors in the face of impending death. To prevent "secondary suffering,"[5] family members also need support and encouragement to develop new ways of interacting and to express their thoughts and feelings. The patient may require a degree of support that family members cannot provide because of their own pain and stress. It is then necessary to develop other support networks for the patient.

Family members must determine an empathic way of relating to the patient without compromising the patient's own needs and sense of self-esteem. This requires seeing the patient as a living person, not as an object or as a disease, and allowing the patient to make decisions or otherwise maintain control to the extent possible and desired.

NEED FOR SPECIAL INTERVENTION

Changes in family functioning, the family system's inability to make decisions, or lack of flexibility within the system to allow for role changes so that new decision-makers can emerge are clues to the need for special intervention. Similarly, serious dysfunction may be signaled by premature use of the past tense in reference to the patient, changes in the family's usual style of communication, or contradictions between verbal and nonverbal behavior. Unexpressed anger may emerge in hostile, nonverbal ways or may be projected onto caregivers and others.

The style of "waiting for death" is a particularly acute problem which manifests itself differently in every family. The family's long-range plans are postponed, and short-range plans are often abandoned. The disease itself can become the central focus of the family's life, as can the patient's anticipated death. Family members may feel angry at the patient for not dying on time. A family may experience waiting, followed by an abatement of the physical crisis and then by waiting again. This anger ought not be repressed or denied. As uncomfortable as it may seem to admit its true cause, this is preferable to allowing the anger to persist unexpressed. Family members should be reassured that such feelings are normal.

Although hospital caregivers have become increasingly aware of the psychosocial needs of patients and families, family members as well as patients may feel helpless and out of control when the patient is cared for in a hospital. Their ability to impact upon the situation is limited both by the institutional environment and by the finality of the disease. Anxiety levels are increased even further by the day-to-day uncertainty of the physical illness.

Family therapy is appropriate for the family that wants to make changes in its level of functioning and is unable to do so without external assistance. The therapist can assist family members to discuss feelings of frustration, anger, and love with one another. Not every family requires or benefits from family therapy; many families are capable of handling crises without special outside intervention. Where appropriate, family therapy provides a supportive and nonjudgmental context in which feelings can be expressed and change facilitated. The family therapist assists interactions and encourages communication among family members. The patient should be included in this process; it is helpful for the family to be together and important not to create an artificial or premature separation from the patient.

ISSUES IN FAMILY THERAPY

Families can be identified on a continuum of emotional closeness (enmeshment) to emotional distance (disengagement) of its members. The family's location on this continuum is observed in its patterns of interaction—in other words, do individual members maintain separate identities from one another, or is the blending inappropriately complete? A family that is enmeshed to the extent that its members speak for one another and read one another's minds tends to be a family in which others make decisions for the ill member. The family therapist in this case directs members to speak for themselves and does not allow mind reading.

Assisting families at the other extreme of the emotional-closeness continuum is more problematic. Disengaged families should be approached with an effort to evolve increased closeness, if desired by the family. Skilled intervention is required to determine if and how family members should be encouraged to risk such intimacy. An objective of family therapy is direct, open communication, enabling all family members to think and speak for themselves.

The previously noted flexible/rigid dichotomy, analogous here to an open or closed family system, is also applicable to the family's reaction to family therapy. The caregiver needs to be aware of the family's willingness to accept an outsider into its system. The capacity of the family system to do so depends on family members' cultural backgrounds and societal roles, and on how these roles have been interpreted and incorporated by the family unit.

Some families incorporate outsiders into their system easily; others find outsiders unacceptable, particularly during periods of stress. The facility with which an outsider is accepted regulates how much and what kind of family intervention the therapist can provide. For the family with a rigid, closed system, the therapist may join the system by assisting initially with concrete services, such as financial matters. This enables the family to develop a degree of trust and to allow an outsider to assist with emotional and interpersonal family issues.

Family therapists should respond to what the family actually brings to the situation. The family therapist must not act from a predetermined frame of reference. The level of crisis should be assessed on the basis of the family's structure and its developmental history. What constitutes a crisis for one person or family does not necessarily constitute a crisis for another.

The patient must not be treated as a temporary or provisional family member. Premature separation may be evidenced by family members' desire to be done with the problems that the patient presents and to get on with their lives. This problem needs attention; it will cause difficulties for the patient and serious problems for family members later on.

Terminal illness in a family member will inevitably preempt other aspects of life. However, as many areas of the family's existence as possible should remain intact. The patient should be encouraged to maintain self-care as long as possible, including dressing, grooming, feeding, and participating in decision making. This will increase the patient's sense of independence and self-esteem. The sense of "normal family life" must be preserved to the fullest extent possible. The illness should be placed into the perspective of the normal lifestyle of the family and not allowed to define or control the family.

The patient should be encouraged to engage in sexual activity to the extent possible and desired by both partners. This may mean redefining sexuality in order to fit physical capabilities and emotional interests. Often, just being physically close to a loved one provides satisfaction for both individuals.

Often serious illness brings the extended family together, with rarely-seen relatives visiting and offering assistance. When this does not occur, the family therapist should gather the extended, multi-generational family together to help the network develop as a support system. The purpose of the extended family meeting is to open communications among family members and to settle unresolved issues between the patient and others. This should decrease the patient's anxiety level and create a more open system for all family members. A subsequent session of the group may be needed because participants often experience a letdown after the initial session where many historical issues have surfaced. Participants also need the opportunity to return to their own roles.

SEPARATION

I give you up a little bit in my free-fall experience. But at the same time I don't want you to give me up. Maybe that's selfish—maybe this is how a dying person expresses his selfishness—that I want you to stay with me even if I am falling away from you.[6]

This kind of separation may be essential for the patient, but it can be devastating to the family that does not understand the patient's needs for gradual withdrawal. Like the patient quoted above, the dying patient may have strong personal needs to separate and may move away from the family. As one member disengages, the family system becomes unbalanced. The family system then responds in some way in an effort to reestablish a state of homeostasis. If the system is unable to reestablish its homeostasis in a natural way, it needs assistance toward restructuring so that it does not become dysfunctional. If the system was dysfunctional when the patient was living, it will remain this way unless change takes place. Restructuring for some families may require the intervention of a therapist who guides the family to change and to surmount the crisis of death.

THE BEREAVED FAMILY

We stood in the hallway crying,
hugging, once in awhile laughing . . .

The center of our world, on which
we'd all been focused for so long,
had suddenly been taken away. We
were swaying dizzily around the edges,
holding on to each other, feeling tears
on each other's cheeks, not knowing how
to let go.[7]

Regardless of what the family has experienced throughout the diagnosis and illness, and despite preparation for the death, the impact of the event itself usually is more overwhelming than had been expected. The full weight of the loss may not be experienced for days or weeks and, as the reality sets in, family members need to be reassured that the sense of loss and feelings of depression are normal. Homeostasis once again is shaken and the family strives to realign roles and to re-focus emotional energies. Bereavement (see Chapter 10), a state of mourning and grief, may continue for well over a year for those most closely attached to the lost person, and at some level it may never end. However, the space occupied by the dead person in the survivor's life should become increasingly small.

Responses to the death of a family member depend on the structure of the family system, on how the family has handled the illness, on the level of communication among family members, and on each individual's social and psychologic characteristics and relationship with the deceased. The circumstances of the death, and the survivor's age, sex, ability to handle stress, and capacity to establish new relationships play a role in the bereavement process.[8] The way that individuals and family systems have experienced and handled separation and loss at other times impacts on how they manage the current situation. Individuals, family subsystems, or the family unit as a whole benefit from the intervention of a family therapist at this time.

Often the experience of emotional isolation extends beyond that of social isolation. Family therapists assist family members to create new affectional bounds and encourage them to form and solidify attachments to others. The goal is not to replace the lost person; this is impossible. In this sense, grieving is never finished. Rather, the aim is to deal with disorganization, despair, and numbness and to assist with the acceptance of and adjustment to the reality of the death.

REFERENCES

1. Andolfi, M.: Family Therapy: An Interactional Approach. New York, Plenum Publishing Corp., 1979.
2. Minuchin, S., and Fishman, H.C.: Family Therapy Techniques. Cambridge, Harvard University Press, p. 11, 1981.
3. Cassileth, B.R., and Hamilton, J.N.: The family with cancer. *In* The Cancer Patient: Social and Medical Aspects of Care. Philadelphia, Lea & Febiger, 1979.
4. Henderson, E.: An approach to the patient with an incurable disease. *In* Psychosocial Aspects of Terminal Care. Edited by B. Schoenberg, A.C. Carr, D. Peretz, and A.H. Kutscher. New York, Columbia University Press, 1972.
5. Weisman, A.D.: Care and comfort of the dying. *In* The Patient, Death and the Family. Edited by S. Troup, and W.A. Green. New York, Charles Scribner and Son, 1974.
6. Smith, J.K.: Free Fall. Valley Forge, Pennsylvania, Judson Press, 1975.
7. Lund, D.: Eric. New York, Dell, p. 10, 1975.
8. Bowlby, J.: Attachment and Loss. Vol. III. New York, Basic Books, 1980.

Chapter 10

Bereavement Care

Arnold Feldman

Bereavement means loss. As such, bereavement and response to it are relevant concerns not only for surviving family members, but also for patients and caregivers, each of whom experiences loss of a particular kind. The term "grief" encompasses those feelings, emotions, and physical symptoms that often accompany an important loss. "Grief work," or mourning, refers to the fact that individuals go through a process of grieving, of experiencing and re-experiencing loss, and ideally, of working through that loss in order to go on to function in a reasonably comfortable way.

SYMPTOMS OF GRIEF

Many of the symptoms or reactions that occur in grieving not only are painful in and of themselves, but also can cause concern in the bereaved about the appropriateness of their reactions. Many people worry that they might not be grieving the "right way" and wonder whether their feelings and responses are "normal." Believing that one sees the dead person, excessive anger, and a sense of irritation with others, often with those who are trying to help, are common examples of reactions that are doubly distressing because the sorrow and despair are compounded by the terrifying sense of loss of rational mental functioning. It is reassuring to the bereaved to learn that their responses are not bizarre or inappropriate.

Pine's and Aronson's term, "the fallacy of uniqueness,"[1] can be applied meaningfully to many situations, including bereavement. "The fallacy of uniqueness" refers to the belief that one is alone and unusual in experiencing distressing feelings and thoughts. That sense, in and of itself, is disturbing. The ability to recognize that one's feelings are common engenders the comfort of knowing that one is functioning within the context of broad human experience.

Anger at having been abandoned by the loved one is a common reaction. Often the bereaved's anger is displaced onto caretakers, and health professionals' efforts are greeted with hostility. Those of us who work with the bereaved must understand that a common underlying cause for the anger is guilt over unresolved issues in the relationship with the loved one.

Most people who suffer a loss find themselves experiencing one or more of the following symptoms: tightness in the throat; heaviness in the chest; an empty feeling in the stomach; diminished appetite; difficulty in concentrating and in completing tasks; and difficulty in sleeping. Other common responses include recurrent dreams about the lost person, restlessness, aimlessness, a sense of isolation and loneliness, frequent mood changes, crying at unexpected times, neglecting one's own health, preoccupation with the life of the deceased, and a need to tell and retell the experience of the loved one's death.

Basic to many symptoms of grief is the fact that survivors continue to focus most of their attention on the person who has died, while retreating from the real world. In the mind of the bereaved, the important person becomes the object of thought; hence the dreaming, the repetitive conversation, the expectation of seeing the dead person in familiar places, and the diminished interest in self and in others.

The need to tell and retell the experience of the death is pressing. A story by Chekov, "The Cabman," beautifully conveys the intensity of this need. In Chekov's tale, an old man who is the driver of a horse-drawn cab tries to tell each fare that his son has died. The story describes how the passengers respond, and although each reacts differently, they all react with utter disinterest. Thus, the fares react jovially, change the subject, or ignore what the cabman has said. The story follows the old man through his day at work and then, as he brings his horse into the stable and unhitches him from the cab, he goes to the horse and says, "You know, my son died today."

The importance of talking about one's grief and the problems that can arise when one fails to do so are captured by Shakespeare in Macbeth. Malcolm says to Macduff:

Give sorrow words; the grief that does
not speak whispers the o'er-fraught
heart and bids it break.

We must emphasize to survivors the need to talk, because some tend to avoid uncomfortable feelings, to protect themselves against experiencing the distress that comes with the talking. However, it is universally held that the failure to share grief increases the risk of serious emotional problems.

The classic study of this subject, still relevant and instructive, is a 1944 article by Eric Lindemann.[2] Lindemann was a psychiatrist at Massachusetts General Hospital at the time of the Coconut Grove fire, in which many people were killed. Much of his work on grieving and on the need for grief work emerged from his study of Coconut Grove survivors. He found that those people who were able to tolerate experiencing the extreme distress, the sadness, the guilt, and the pain, and who were able to talk about their loss, eventually managed to work through the grief and go on with their lives.

As Lindemann explains, the goal of grief work is emancipation from the deceased and formation of new relationships. He hypothesizes that if the grief work is not accomplished, emancipation cannot occur, and one will remain suspended in unresolved grief. His work and that of others suggest that people who experience either no grief or delayed grief have a higher incidence of maladaptive behavior.

PATHOLOGIC GRIEF

Pathologic or dysfunctional grief can take several forms, and it usually is expressed as an extreme of "normal" symptomatology. The common symptom of assuming the loved one's mannerisms, traits, or other aspects of identity, for example, can vary from the relatively benign to the pathologic. For instance, a colleague suddenly noted, sometime after his father's death, that his handwriting had changed and that, unconsciously, he had assumed his father's penmanship. Other people adopt the gait or hobbies of the dead person. Psychologically, these behaviors are ways of retaining some part of the deceased within one's self. One takes on that part and gains a constant reminder or memorial through identification. It is a way of not letting go that is not maladaptive.

Identification also can manifest itself pathologically, as the following example illustrates. A 45-year-old woman developed severe chest pain shortly after her husband died from a heart attack. In this woman the electrocardiogram and blood tests remained normal and the primary etiology of her symptoms clearly was psychologic. Lindemann's article on grief describes a man whose electrocardiogram actually became abnormal following the heart attack death of his spouse.[2] In his case, the extent of the physiologic response to his emotional identification with his wife was manifest objectively.

Delayed grief is another pathologic reaction. A frequent expression of this phenomenon is exemplified by a 42-year-old man who developed intense feelings of sadness and grief, for the first time, 20 years after the death of his mother who had died at the age of 42. Events such as this are known as the "anniversary reaction," wherein the impact of the loss recurs or is felt for the first time at significant points in time.

Survivors who have denied the terminal nature of a loved one's illness, despite attempts at intervention, tend to do badly, experiencing great difficulty during bereavement. If the specter of the death was so frightening as to exclude anticipatory grief, the coping skills of such individuals tend to be inadequate for the challenges that lie ahead, and problems can be anticipated. Chronic grief, another maladaptive expression, is seen in people who cannot conclude the grieving process and who remain life-long grievers.

Parkes's work, *Bereavement: Studies of Grief in Adult Life*, contains a review of psychologic and physical illnesses that occur following loss.[3] Most of these studies report an incidence of physical illness and death in the surviving spouse within a year following the loss that is significantly higher than expected. How this occurs is not yet entirely clear, although a sequence of events involving depression of the immune system or altered autonomic function has been postulated.

The response of animals to the loss of a mate is revealing: they continue to search for the dead mate. Geese, for example, will fly greater distances each day and give a specific cry in an effort to find the lost mate. Eventually, their patterns of flight become confused until the ordered pattern dissipates and the search becomes frantically confused.

This behavior among geese is relevant because, in humans as well as in other animals, searching behavior typically has a rationale. We search for "lost" objects and people until we find them.

In response to the death of a loved one, as Parkes notes, the survivor retains that instinct to search, but part of him knows that there is no point in searching, that the continued search is irrational. This may explain the restlessness and the pacing seen in the bereaved. It is as though a part of the individual needs to continue looking while another part recognizes the futility of that instinctual urge. Thus, there is movement, but no goal; the ultimate goal, being irrational, is inhibited.

In pathologic grief, although not in most grieving processes, significant suicidal ideation may occur. At times the thought that "I don't want to go on living without my spouse" may engulf the bereaved, but it is rarely pursued. Freud's "Mourning and Melancholia" compares symptoms of bereavement to those of depression. Freud saw the two conditions as sharing many symptoms: profoundly painful dejection; decreased interest in the outside world; diminished capacity to love; and severely inhibited activity. He describes the loss of self-esteem as the crucial difference between mourning and depression, but this is more a quantitative than a qualitative distinction. In the broad spectrum of grief reaction, the individual often experiences a loss of self-esteem and some feelings of guilt. If these become marked and severe, leaving the individual feeling worthless and overridden by guilt, one has entered the sphere of pathologic guilt.

This kind of grief is comparable to severe depressive reaction rather than to bereavement response. The griever typically communicates a sense of great despondency accompanied by a transient loss of desire to continue living. It is always appropriate from a professional perspective to inquire about suicidal ideation; such questioning does *not* precipitate suicide attempts. More lives are saved by asking than by failing to ask. Suicide is the extreme reaction and it does occur, but rarely.

FACTORS THAT INFLUENCE BEREAVEMENT

Loss plays a major role in human growth. Each maturational step is accompanied by a giving up of someone or something. The early separation of the child from its mother, the move from high school to college, and work changes from job advancement all involve some degree of loss. Previous adaptation to loss is the best predictor of future coping. People who have lost parents when they were children are at particularly high risk of responding poorly to the death of a spouse, and those who have experienced a significant previous loss that they were unable to work through are at risk of maladaptive response.

One's relationship to the deceased, the timing of the death, and the support system of the survivors all influence the bereaved's response to death. Adults, by and large, do not react to the death of a parent as intensely as they respond to the death of a spouse or child.

Although death is rarely welcome, its occurrence is less shocking to the survivors when it is time-appropriate. When someone dies in his or her eighties, after a full life, survivors respond differently than they would to the death of a thirty-year-old. Intrinsic notions of "fairness" or "rightness," in part, define one's response, as does the extent to which survivors are prepared for the death. The support system in place at the time of loss is a strong predictor of how well survivors will handle the death. Close friends and family are needed at this time.

ANTICIPATORY GRIEF

How long after the onset of illness did the person die? Was it a prolonged illness lasting, say, more than six months; was death sudden; or was the duration of illness for a period of time in between? This is important because the bereaved's response to the death may correlate with the amount of preparatory time involved. The problem with sudden death is clear: survivors have had no time to prepare for the loss, and the numbness and shock are more profound than reactions that follow prolonged illness.

Anticipatory grief refers to the fact that people can begin to grieve prior to the death of the patient. Anticipatory grief can ease the pain, if, for example, a husband and wife can begin to talk about what is happening during the terminal stages of disease, to share feelings, and to experience closeness. Both the dying person and the family member can thereby begin to work through some of the feelings of loss, sadness, and anger.

Anticipatory grief can reduce the sudden impact—the shock of loss—and it can help achieve a meaningful time together for the patient's loved one as well as for the patient himself. The dying person is grieving too, but his is a much greater grief because he will lose everything. The survivors will lose an important person, but they will have other people and life itself left. One of the most distressing aspects of death is precisely that, through it, every-thing and everyone are lost. This finality and aloneness contribute to religious notions of an afterlife in which one rejoins loved ones, a compensatory concept that deals with a universal dread.

One of the dangers of anticipatory grief is the possibility that family and friends will become emotionally detached prior to the person's death. This has been a problem for some parents of chil-dren with terminal stage leukemia, who had been given a precise prognosis regarding the amount of time left to the child. They started to grieve and, as grief work induced detachment, they became emancipated from the dying child. The child who lived much beyond the anticipated time became psychologically dead to other family members.

Lindemann describes this as a frequent occurrence during the Second World War, when relatives of men sent to the front would experience anticipatory grief because their men were not expected to return. When these sons and husbands did survive to return home, their families found it extremely difficult to relate to them because, for them, the unexpectedly returned soldiers were dead.

There is another unfortunate and ironic effect of living beyond one's "allotted time": a sense among patients, families, and care-givers that the patient is living "too long," that he has failed to die on time. When illness extends beyond an expected period, it is felt to "drag on" inappropriately, and family members, physi-cians, and nurses begin to feel overburdened and to wish for the death of the patient. This in turn creates expanded guilt, which fires anger and more guilt. Sometimes this situation is the inevi-table consequence of an unusual course of illness. Often, however, it can be avoided if the physician does not orient the patient and family to expect death in a particular number of weeks or months.

ASSISTING THE BEREAVED

Psychotherapists can work effectively with pathologic grief, delayed grief, or the absence of grief; for example, they can assist the survivor to experience normal grieving through which eman-cipation from the deceased can be achieved. Laymen can also do much to assist survivors who are dealing with the non-pathologic pain of bereavement. Immediately following the loss, when the survivor's reaction is best characterized by numbness and immobility, the kind of help needed is practical, such as assistance with the chores of everyday living. A period of numbness typically precedes the need to talk. In the period immediately after the loss, helping to prepare meals or performing household chores is of great value to the bereaved. Sympathetic listening is critically needed later on.

The role of those working with the bereaved is to supplement rather than supplant support systems that already exist in the bereaved person's environment. We must avoid attempting to replace support systems. Illich speaks of traditional American institutions such as family and church having weakened substantially and become less available and helpful than they once were.[4] People now tend to turn to the health professions for help once available elsewhere. To what extent is intervention by health caregivers appropriate? In the case of death and bereavement, care need be taken not to undermine inadvertently or weaken existing sources of support in the family or in the larger environment by providing too much direction and assistance.

A related dilemma especially relevant to care of the terminally ill and the bereaved is the risk for health professionals of over-identification with patients or survivors. Frequently, we are beset by the feeling that more must be done than we are realistically able to accomplish. Working with dying patients often revives one's own experiences with loss, and one tends to try to work through one's own problems and previous losses while dealing with the patient and family.

Compassion is prerequisite for work with the terminally ill but, as Cassem has clearly noted,[5] we pay a price for compassion. We constantly establish relationships in which we play a caring and compassionate role, only to experience consecutive losses with the emotional impact that loss entails. A perspective that one is working with people during this particular time in their lives, rather than working with the dying, assists us to work effectively and with minimal personal disruption, but the natural human tendency to mourn loss remains a major difficulty for caregivers.

REFERENCES

1. Pines, A.M., Aronson, E., and Kafry, D.: Burnout: From Tedium to Personal Growth. New York, Free Press, 1980.

2. Lindemann, E.: The symptomatology and management of acute grief. Am. J. Psychiatry, *101*:141-147, 1944.
3. Parkes, C.M.: Bereavement: Studies of Grief in Adult Life. New York, International Universities Press, 1973.
4. Illich, I.: Medical Nemesis. New York, Bantam Books, 1977.
5. Cassem, N.H.: The dying patient. *In* Massachusetts General Hospital Handbook of General Hospital Psychiatry. Edited by T.P. Hackett, and N.H. Cassem. St. Louis, C.V. Mosby, 1978.

Chapter 11

Nutritional Care

Lon O. Crosby

The relationship between malnutrition and cancer has been known for thousands of years, and was described in the Hippocratic era.[1] The first major research on this interaction was conducted in the 1930s by Warren, who linked the severity of cancer to resultant nutritional status.[2] In the following decade, many studies investigated potential means of reversing the iatrogenic and tumor-induced malnutrition associated with metastatic disease. These attempts were uniformly unsuccessful, and clinical interest in this field waned rapidly. Few scientists maintained interest in nutritional problems as the development of improved surgical techniques, antibiotics, anesthetic agents, chemotherapy, and radiation therapy enabled major advances in cancer treatment and overshadowed concern with nutritional sequelae.

During this same period, however, other researchers investigated the impact of nutritional status on the outcome of surgical procedures. The work of Ravdin, Cuthbertson, Rhoads, and others documented the relationship between malnutrition, impaired wound healing, and postoperative infection.[3] The metabolic abnormalities induced by malnutrition and by the catabolic effects of surgery stimulated research during the 1940s and 1950s on enteral and parenteral administration of nutrients.[4] Early attempts to maintain surgical patients in positive energy and protein balance failed, however, because it was impossible at that time to deliver sufficient nutrients without undue complications.

It was not until 1967 that technical problems associated with the administration of nutrients were resolved. Dudrick, Wilmore,

Vars, and Rhoads documented normal growth in puppies following application of intravenous hyperalimentation.[5,6] This technique was applied to humans shortly thereafter, and is considered to be a landmark of modern medicine. The development and application of total parenteral nutrition, as it is now called, laid the foundation for major improvements in clinical care. Subsequent advances in this area and in enteral nutrition enabled physicians to extend the life of many patients, and simultaneously raised a number of moral and ethical questions about the use of nutritional support in cancer patients. As is true of other advances in medical care, such as cardiac and pulmonary assistance and dialysis, nutritional support techniques can maintain life long after qualitatively meaningful life exists. The ethical and moral issues surrounding implementation and continuation of nutritional support for the terminal cancer patient remain troublesome. The decision to provide nutritional support requires an understanding of the totality of the specific patient's medical and personal status.[7]

STARVATION: A MODEL OF SEVERE MALNUTRITION

The effects of malnutrition in terminal cancer patients can be as severe as those observed in conditions of starvation. A great deal is known about the physiologic changes that occur in starvation from studies that do not involve patients with cancer. The effects of starvation are best described by defining physiologic changes in body water, fat, protein, and cell mass. Body cell mass is the sum weight of work-perfoming tissue in the body and is directly related to energy metabolism.[4] Regardless of whether starvation is caused directly by reduced food intake or indirectly by disease or treatment, the results are similar. Body weight, fat, protein, and cell mass decrease, and total body water increases (with intracellular water decreasing and extracellular water increasing).

There are three phases of starvation. The point at which each phase is reached depends on the relative degree of nutrient deprivation and on the confounding effects of disease and/or stress. The first phase, which occurs during the initial week of reduced food intake, results in a rapid loss of body protein with minimal loss of fat stores. The second phase occurs over the next three to six weeks, and represents the body's attempt to conserve body proteins through markedly increased utilization of fat. The third stage results in massive alterations in metabolism as the body metabolizes ketones derived from proteins and lipids. This adaptation causes fluid conservation, sodium retention, and major shifts in intracellular fluids which result in the edema-anasarca state frequently seen in starvation. In the third stage, an unstressed patient with no confounding disease loses from 180 to 300 grams of muscle tissue per day (an average of 6 to 10 grams of nitrogen and approximately 150 to 250 grams of fat are burned per day, equivalent to 1350–2250 calories). The total daily weight loss, therefore, approximates 500 grams or approximately 1 pound. Active disease can double this rate of loss.[8–10]

The rate of mobilization and of fat and protein utilization during starvation are determined by the amount of energy required to maintain body temperature and basal activity of the heart, respiratory muscles, nerves, and glands. To these basal requirements are added exercise needs for whatever external muscle work is performed. For cancer patients, the energy requirements of tissue repair, stress, and the costs of the body's defenses against tumor growth must be added. In addition, many tumors are thought to excrete substances that decrease the host's efficiency of energy utilization, whether the energy is derived from food or from body stores.[11] Knowledgeable nutritional support can reverse these changes or prevent their progression.[12–13]

THE INCIDENCE OF MALNUTRITION IN CANCER PATIENTS

Studies of malnutrition in hospitalized patients by Blackburn and Butterworth in the early 1970s refocused attention on malnutrition generally and on cancer patients in particular.[14] To understand malnutrition in cancer patients, it helps to review malnutrition in the general population. In the United States, the incidence of severe malnutrition such as occurs in kwashiorkor, scurvy, or beriberi is low. However, the situation is markedly different when biochemical indicators of nutritional status are examined.

Published data indicate the presence of hypoalbuminemia (apparent protein deficiency) in 5 to 7% of individuals over the age of 59. For the vitamins studied (riboflavin, thiamine, vitamin A, and vitamin C), between 5 and 10% of individuals have low or deficient levels. Mineral deficiencies (iodine and iron) occur in 5 and 15% of the population, respectively. Age, sex, race, weight, and income all contribute to the incidence of biochemical malnutrition. Most disturbing is the fact that over 50% of individuals over the age of 59 are deficient in one or more of those nutrients that have been investigated. If all known nutrients were studied, the incidence of malnutrition would prove substantially higher. Even in white high-income groups, the incidence of malnutrition as just defined is 25%.[15] Unfortunately, no similar comprehensive studies have been conducted with cancer patients. However, available data reveal, not unexpectedly, a much higher incidence of malnutrition among patients presenting for cancer therapy than among the general population.[16] Against this background, the finding that malnutrition is the primary cause of death in cancer patients is not surprising.[2]

NUTRITION INFORMATION NEEDED FOR DECISION-MAKING

A rational and viable nutrition intervention plan for the terminal cancer patient requires acquiring considerable information in order to assess nutritional status and nutritional requirements.[17,18] Anthropometric assessment should determine, at a minimum, height; current, usual, and ideal body weight; and triceps skinfold and midarm muscle circumference. Biochemical assessment should at least determine serum albumin, iron binding capacity, total protein, complete blood count, and delayed hypersensitivity response skin tests. Ideally, current nutrient intake may be determined from a dietary diary or from hospital records over a seven-day period. If this is impossible, macro-nutrient intake can be estimated by dietary recall or by questioning about food frequency. Family members and nursing staff are helpful resources in acquiring information about nutrient intake. Nutrient intake history also should include documentation of changes in the patient's food preferences and gustatory/olfactory responses, satiety levels, and appetite.

In addition to dietary history, the evaluation of iatrogenic nutritional deficiencies due to medication effects and to nutrient/treatment interactions deserves special emphasis. Information about confounding dietary prescriptions (e.g., low sodium diet for hypertension) and problems with constipation, diarrhea, and urination should be sought. Integrating all of these data allows determination of the probable cause(s) of existing cancer cachexia

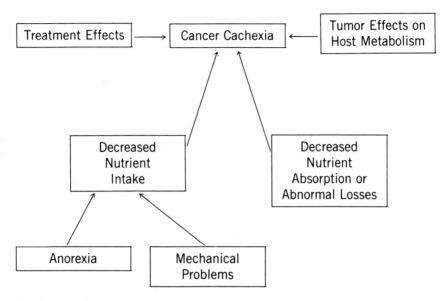

Fig. 11–1. Potential causes of cancer cachexia.

(Fig. 11–1), or evaluation of the likelihood of impending cachexia. Once the degree of malnutrition is documented and the probable causes defined, a plan for supportive intervention can be developed.

Nutritional support should aim for a series of short-term, beneficial goals that will impact usefully on the patient and on the patient's care. Relevant goals have multiple dimensions, including increasing fluid intake, controlling diarrhea, increasing caloric intake, facilitating meal preparation for the spouse, and increasing the number of meals offered to the patient, for example. Successful implementation of a series of efforts aimed at short-term goals should result in long-term nutrition improvement or maintenance. Efforts are directed sequentially toward resolving medical/nutritional problems, and then toward preventing nutritional complications.

METHODS OF NUTRITIONAL SUPPORT

Several methods increase nutrient intake in cancer patients,[19-21] as shown in Table 11–1. These procedures require knowledge and expertise on the part of the health care community. The general approach is to use the *least invasive* procedure that will suffice to maintain the cancer patient's nutritional status. Each of

TABLE 11–1. Methods of Nutritional Intervention.

I. *Medical Intervention to Avoid or Minimize Complications*
  A. Medication to control treatment and/or disease side effects, e.g., nausea, vomiting, diarrhea, pain
  B. Appetite stimulants
  C. Provision for artificial saliva, dental prosthesis, necessary digestive enzymes
  D. Medication to control depression, anxiety, etc.
II. *Indirect Intervention*
  A. Selection and/or alteration of foods to increase acceptability
  B. Counseling
    1. Informal
    2. Formal
  C. Psychologic support
    1. General intervention
    2. Behavior modification
III. *Direct Intervention*
  A. Enteral supplementation
    1. Incomplete diet
    2. Complete diet
  B. Total enteral nutrition
    1. Naso-intestinal tube
    2. Gastrostomy
    3. Jejunostomy
  C. Total parenteral nutrition
    1. Peripheral vein
    2. Central vein

these intervention techniques is reviewed below, as each is applicable potentially to the terminally ill cancer patient.

An important aspect of improving the nutritional status of terminal cancer patients is the control of symptoms induced by the disease and by the treatment. Sometimes an effective pain control regimen or the application of agents to control nausea, vomiting, or diarrhea may suffice to increase food intake to an acceptable level. These approaches may obviate the need for any direct or indirect nutritional intervention.

Indirect nutritional intervention has been used intuitively by the lay population for years. Giving special treats to a child during an illness is one example. This approach remains an important inducement for increased food intake. The situation is more complex with cancer patients, however, because both the disease and its therapy affect taste and smell perception. Food preference surveys show that changes in consumption result. The most common of these are the development of dislike for the taste of meat and the preference for spicy, Oriental-type foods.

In a terminal care setting, informal counseling and encouragement can be powerful tools for achieving increased food intake.

This is especially true when those caring for the patient, including family, physicians, and staff, offer support and encouragement toward improved eating habits. Formal counseling can be provided by many members of the health care team, although usually this responsibility is assigned to a dietician. The collection of intake and preference data, the development of a nutritional prescription, and the mutual review of progress toward established goals also are necessary and effective.

Psychologic support may help increase nutrient intake by ameliorating some of the stresses faced by the patient. One such means is the intervention of a social worker to provide general support and to help resolve practical problems. If necessary, a psychologist or psychiatrist may be called in to assist. Behavior modification techniques also may be helpful.

Although no controlled clinical trials have been performed to document the efficacy of indirect intervention techniques, clinical observations suggest that they are effective. They are less so under conditions of severe malnutrition and nutrition-related complications.

Direct intervention techniques are of two general types. The first, enteral supplementation, relies upon the patient's voluntary cooperation to increase nutrient intake and assumes the presence of medical intervention to minimize or prevent complications of the disease and treatment. The second, total enteral or total parenteral nutrition, removes control of nutrient intake from the patient. Nutrients are infused directly into the intestinal tract or vasculature. Several commercial products used for total enteral nutrition and enteral supplementation are listed in Table 11–2.

Enteral supplements can be used in a variety of situations in which nutrient intake is temporarily or chronically reduced, but in which additional oral intake is feasible. Enteral supplements frequently increase nutrient calories and protein to acceptable levels. A variety of commercial oral supplements are available as listed in Table 11–3.

Relatively simple modifications in meal preparation can be attempted, including the use of double or triple strength milk (adding powdered milk to regular milk) in order to increase protein intake, or the use of additional fats in cooking to increase calorie intake.

The selection of total enteral nutrition versus total parenteral nutrition is based upon the integrity and function of the gastrointestinal tract. If nutrient absorption and intestinal tract function

TABLE 11–2. Selected Commercial Products Available for Total Enteral Nutrition and Enteral Supplementation.

A. *Intact Protein—Containing Lactose*
   Carnation: CIB
   Cutter: Formula 2, Nutri-1000
   Doyle: Compleat-B, Meritene Liquid
   Mead Johnson: Sustacal
   Organon: Vitaneed

B. *Intact Protein/Protein Isolates—Low or Free of Lactose*
   Cutter: Nutri-1000 LF
   Doyle: Precision Isotonic, Precision HN, Precision LR
   Mead Johnson: Isocal, Portagen, ProSobee
   Ross: Ensure, Ensure Plus, Isomil, Osmolite

C. *Hydrolyzed Protein/Amino Acids—Low or Free of Lactose*
   Cutter: Vipep
   Eaton: Vivonex, Vivonex HN
   Mead Johnson: Flexical, Nutramigen, Pregestimil
   Ross: Vital

are normal, total enteral support is the preferred route. The commercial products listed in Table 11–4 utilize intact proteins, protein isolates, protein hydrolysates, and crystalline amino acids.

Long-term support of cancer patients by total parenteral and total enteral nutrition is feasible. Implementation of intensive nutritional support requires the availability of a specialized nutrition support service comprised of physicians, nurses, dieticians, and pharmacists. Intensive nutritional support for cancer patients is safe and efficacious, if provided by individuals trained in its application.

DECISION-MAKING IN TERMINAL ILLNESS

The general consensus is that intensive nutritional support should not be attempted with patients from whom intensive medical support has been withdrawn. However, every case is different, and each patient requires individual consideration. The following case histories illustrate the clinical and ethical dilemmas faced by health professionals in this regard.

CASE 1

A 36-year-old woman with ovarian cancer and abdominal metastases had exhausted all effective treatment. She had been supported by total parenteral nutrition throughout sev-

TABLE 11–3. Selected Commercial Products for Oral Supplementation.*

Company	Product	Function/Source
Beecham Laboratories	Hycal	Carbohydrate
Navco	Pro-Mix	Protein
Control Drugs	EMF	Protein
Doyle	Citrotein	Protein, vitamins
	Controlyte	Calories
General Mills	Cal Power	Carbohydrate
	High Pen Protein	Protein
Organon	Microlipid	Lipid
	Sustacal	Carbohydrate
	Sustacal Powder	Carbohydrate
Mead Johnson	Sustacal Pudding	Complete supplement
	Lofenalac	Metabolic complications
	Phenylfree	Metabolic complications
Lederle	Geural	Protein/calorie
Mead Johnson	Casec	Protein
	Lonalac	Protein/calorie
	Lytren	Calorie
	MCT Oil	Lipid
	Probana	Protein, diarrhea control
Ross	Pedialyte	Calorie/electrolyte
	Polycose	Carbohydrate
Upjohn	Lipomul-Oral	Lipid
	Liprotein	Protein/calorie
McGaw	Amin-Aid	Metabolic complications
	Hepatic Aid	Metabolic complications

*These products can be combined together or with other food products to meet nutrition needs. Note that many grocery store products, such as instant breakfast products and liquid dietetic solutions, can be used effectively in enteral nutrition regimens.

eral previous treatment regimens. This support was discontinued during the last chemotherapy cycle because of treatment complications. The oncologists predicted a four to six months survival with palliative chemotherapy and intensive nutritional intervention, or two to four weeks survival with no intervention. It was felt that the patient's quality of life would be high until death became imminent. The patient had three young children with whom she wanted to spend as much time as possible. This patient was placed on home parenteral nutrition (a form of total parenteral nutrition), and was taught to self-administer nutrient solutions through a permanent right

TABLE 11–4. Selected Commercial Products Available for Total Parenteral Nutrition.

A. *Amino Acid Sources*
   Abbott: Aminosyn
   Cutter: Veinamine
   McGaw: Freamine III, Nephramine
   Travenol: Travasol

B. *Carbohydrate Sources*
   Many companies make 50/70% intravenous dextrose.

C. *Lipid*
   Cutter: Intralipid
   Abbott: Liposyn

D. *Minerals*
   American Quinine: Individual and multiple trace elements (Ca, Cn, and Zn)
   Abbott: Individual (Ca, Cr, Mn, and Zn)
   IMS: Multiple vitamin solution

E. *Vitamins*
   USV: MVI Maintenance, MVI Concentrate, MVI Solution
   Roche: Berocca C
   Abbott: Multi-vitamin additive
   Ascot: MVC solution
   IMS: Multiple vitamin solution

   Many companies make single vitamin solutions for IV/IM use.

atrial catheter. She subsequently spent five months at home prior to death.

CASE 2

A 55-year-old man with metastatic lung cancer was admitted to the intensive care unit for respiratory failure, probable stroke, and sepsis. Total parenteral nutrition was initiated. Nutritional support was discontinued after seven days in accordance with the family's request to discontinue heroic medical efforts.

CASE 3

A 68-year-old woman with breast cancer metastatic to the liver was admitted to the hospital after failing several chemotherapy regimens. She was obviously malnourished (serum albumin of 2.0 g/100 ml and 65% of ideal body weight). She wished to live to experience her 50th wedding anniversary, one month hence. Projected survival was less than one week with no intervention and two to four weeks with palliative therapy and intensive nutritional support. Nutritional support was initiated for this patient, consisting of oral supplements and supplemental infusion of nutrients through a peripheral vein.

CASE 4

A 70-year-old man with unresectable gastric carcinoma had a feeding jejunostomy established with all subsequent nourishment provided by total enteral nutrition. He subsequently failed chemotherapy with evidence of progressive disease. The patient was transferred to a nursing home with a life expectancy of four to six weeks. Nutritional support was continued until the patient's condition deteriorated markedly as a result of tumor growth.

Ultimately, the decision to intervene nutritionally is based on the determination that nutrient intake is inadequate to meet needs and that intervention will improve the patient's quality of life. Under these conditions, the attempt is made to meet caloric needs by introducing carbohydrates and lipids and to meet amino acid requirements by administering protein. If these requirements can be satisfied through a variety of methods, adequate micro-nutrients (vitamins, minerals, and trace elements) are provided easily by administering an oral or intravenous vitamin and mineral mixture.

In considering nutritional support, one must take into account the important role that food plays in everyday life. The provision and consumption of food are social phenomena that involve the atmosphere and circumstances under which nutrients are delivered.[22] As medical treatment programs become more complex and sophisticated, the provision of food and the participation in a nutritional support program often remain the only opportunities for cancer patients and their families to participate in the health care process.[23-25]

OTHER CONSIDERATIONS

Many factors beyond the scope of this chapter also must be considered in the development and maintenance of nutritional care for terminally ill patients. These are described briefly below.

Economic Considerations

To be useful, an intervention program must be economically feasible. Recent changes in Medicaid-Medicare regulations, which now include reimbursement for nutritional supplements, have eased considerably what has been a substantial family burden. Before an intervention scheme is decided upon definitely, the patient's family or a social worker should be consulted to discuss financial considerations.

Legal Issues

Nutritional support of the terminally ill raises many legal questions. Major concerns include patients' rights to adequate nutrition and informed consent issues regarding involuntary feeding when total parenteral or enteral nutrition regimens are considered.

Psychologic Factors

Those charged with developing nutrition regimens for terminally ill cancer patients must recognize the short- and long-term consequences of the proposed plan, including its emotional and social impact. Moreover, the time at which nutritional support is initiated may be critical to its success. For example, early implementation of a nutrition regimen, before overall therapy objectives have been established, can be counterproductive. Once an aggressive nutritional program is begun, withdrawal may have negative prognostic implications for the patient, while later alterations in the patient's status and therapy may render the nutrition regimen inappropriate. Finally, the psychologic import of the nutrition regimen must be recognized. Attention to a patient's nutritional status, particularly when anti-neoplastic therapy has been terminated, demonstrates continuing professional concern and care and thus can decrease the patient's sense of hopelessness and depression.

Malnutrition no longer is an inevitable consequence of metastatic disease and its treatment. However, because current medical technology enables the maintenance of life long after there is any rational hope for improvement, the application of nutritional support modalities always should be consonant with overall medical management objectives. Reasonable patient requests, probable survival duration, and quality of life together must serve as guidelines for the selection, institution, and maintenance of nutritional support. Provision of nutritional support is not an all-or-nothing decision. Rather, use can be made of the many alternatives available and support adjusted as the patient's condition changes. Because the metabolic consequences of malnutrition can and frequently do create complications that adversely affect the patient's existence, nutritional management considerations should be a part of all terminal treatment programs.

REFERENCES

1. Pitot, H.C.: Fundamentals of Oncology. New York, Marcel Dekker, 1978.
2. Warren, S.: The immediate causes of death in cancer. Am. J. Med. Sci., *184*:610–615, 1932.
3. Rhoads, J.E., Bars, H.M., and Dudrick, S.J.: The development of intravenous hyperalimentation. *In* Surgical Clinics of North America. Vol. 61. Edited by B. Cohen. *3*:429-463, 1981.
4. Costa, G.: Hypothetical pathway of nitrogen metabolism. Nature, *188*:549–552, 1960.
5. Dudrick, S.J., Wilmore, D.W., and Vars, H.M.: Long-term parenteral nutrition with growth in puppies and positive nitrogen balance in patients. Surg. Forum, *18*:356–357, 1967.
6. Dudrick, S.J., Wilmore, D.W., Vars, H.M., and Rhoads, J.E.: Long-term total parenteral nutrition and growth, development and positive nitrogen balance. Surgery *64*:134–142, 1968.
7. Brennan, M.F.: Total parenteral nutrition in the cancer patient. New Engl. J. Med., *305*:375–382, 1981.
8. Benedict, F.G.: A study of prolonged fastings. Carnegie Institute of Washington, Publ. 203, 1915.
9. Cahill, G.F.: Starvation in man. New Engl. J. Med., *282*:668–675, 1970.
10. Waterlow, J.C.: Protein nutrition and metabolism in the whole animal. *In* Mammalian Protein Metabolism. Edited by H.N. Munro. New York, Academic Press, 1973.
11. Waterhouse, C.: How tumors affect host metabolism. Ann. N.Y. Acad. Sci., *230*:86–93, 1974.
12. Shizgal, H.M., Spanier, A.H., and Kurtz, R.S.: Effect of parenteral nutrition on body composition in the critically ill patient. Am. J. Surg., *131*:156–161, 1976.
13. Kurtz, R.S., Wood, C.D., and Shizgal, H.M.: Effect of parenteral nutrition on body composition. Surg. Forum, *25*:63–65, 1974.
14. Butterworth, C., and Blackburn, G.: Hospital malnutrition. Nutr. Today, *10*:8–18, 1975.
15. Department of Health, Education and Welfare: Ten State Nutrition Survey. DHEW Publication Numbers 72–8130, 72–8131, 72–8133, 1972.
16. Butterworth, C.E.: Prevalence of vitamin deficiencies in cancer patients as detailed by a multi-phasic biochemical screening procedure. Amer. Coll. of Nutr., 1980; September 8–9 (abstract).

17. Mullen, J., Crosby, L., and Rombeau, J. (Eds.): Surgical Nutrition. Surg. Clin. North Am., *61*:1–761, 1981.
18. Goodhart, R.S., and Shils, M.E.: Modern Nutrition in Health and Disease. Philadelphia, Lea & Febiger, 1980.
19. Conference on Nutrition and Cancer Therapy: Cancer Res., *37*(7) Part 2:2322–2471, 1977.
20. Department of Health, Education and Welfare: Federal and Non-federal Resources for Nutritional Information and Services: A Selected List. *USGPO* 629–94612438, 1979.
21. Department of Health and Human Services: Coping with Cancer: A Resource for the Health Professional. HSS Publication Number 80–2080, 1980.
22. Getz, G.M.: Nutritional services. *In* The Cancer Patient: Social and Medical Aspects of Care. Edited by B.R. Cassileth. Philadelphia, Lea & Febiger, 1979.
23. Dunlop, B.D.: Expanded home-based care for the elderly: solution or pipe dream? Am. J. Public Health, *70*:514–519, 1980.
24. Barckley, V.: Caring for the cancer patient at home. J. Practical Nurs., *24*:24–27 1974.
25. Suski, N.S.: Home consultation for the terminally ill. J. Am. Diet. Assoc., *78*:620–622, 1981.

Chapter 12

Home Care

Joanne Packer-Weiss

In 1859, an Englishman named Mr. William Rathbone developed and established the first plan for utilizing graduate nurses to care for the sick and poor in their homes. Approximately 20 years later the women's branch of the New York City Mission became the first establishment in the United States to hire graduate nurses for the provision of in-home services. The principles and philosophies of this organized activity encompassed both a professional and a spiritual approach to providing care for the sick and poor in their homes.[1]

The first voluntary, nongovernment home health agency was established in Buffalo, New York, in 1885, and this was followed by the development of similar agencies in Philadelphia and Boston one year later. These agencies, begun by lay people, later became what we know today as the visiting nurse associations. Their purpose was to provide care in the home to the sick and to teach family members personal hygiene and other aspects of the care and management of the sick at home. No source of financing existed, and with each visit patients were asked to contribute some part of the cost.[2]

The first official government effort occurred in 1896, when the Los Angeles County Health Department hired graduate nurses to provide care in patients' homes. Meanwhile, visiting nurse associations continued to grow and were established across the United States. Following the Los Angeles model, county health departments became the primary home care agencies in the southwestern portion of the country. In both voluntary and government agencies,

nursing was the first and, for many years, the only discipline involved in providing care in patients' homes. Over time, additional
assistance—social workers, physical therapists, nutritionists,
speech therapists, occupational therapists, home makers, and home
health aids, in that order—was provided, although this was not
available everywhere.[2]

As early as 1909, one major health insurance company realized
the advantage of home care and offered services to some of its
clients. There was little interest generally in this plan of care, and
only one or two other companies utilized any of the services until
the middle 1960s. For almost a century, home care services were
provided throughout the country by a variety of associations, mis-
sions, and agencies. These services then were directed primarily
at the poor. Usage was dramatically affected by Titles 18 and 19
of the federal Social Security Act, which permit reimbursement
for home care services under Medicare and Medicaid respectively.[3]

THE EMERGENCE OF MODERN HOME HEALTH SERVICES

Just as medicine has made advances in the treatment of disease
and nursing has kept pace to provide care to patients treated with
new techniques, the home health care delivery system has expanded to provide multidisciplinary services in the home. The benefits of home health care are basically twofold. First, home care
is a cost-effective means of providing comprehensive health services, particularly in comparison to rapidly escalating, inpatient hospital costs. Second, home health care provides continuity of care
from hospital to home for convalescence, for rehabilitation, or for
terminal care.[4]

Home health nursing is one facet of a coordinated home care
system. In many areas, it has incorporated or replaced visiting
nurse associations. In more than one city, for example, visiting
nurse associations that for years were combined with city health
departments, severed those ties to become independent home
health service affiliates of visiting nurse associations.

Home care services began as an effort to aid the poor; such
services are available now to anyone regardless of socioeconomic
status. A stigma remains, however, that these services still are
for the financially needy. The association between home health
care and hospice probably will reduce that stigma, as will the

financial facts. Home visits are provided by members of a multi-disciplinary team, and few of these visits are free. Most visiting nurse associations or their affiliates, however, serve patients regardless of their ability to pay.[1] Third-party insurers as well as state and federal governments reimburse or pay directly for most home care.[3] Services now are provided by home health agencies that are voluntary, government affiliated, or a combination of both. Most are nonprofit, although increasing numbers of proprietary organizations have entered the home care business.

Today, Medicare is a trend setter for other third-party insurers in determining which services are reimbursable. In the years since Medicare became involved in home care, many new agencies have incorporated themselves into what is called the "Medicare business."[3] Although high quality patient care is a basis for their development, business concerns occasionally and unfortunately supersede their patient orientation.

Home care and hospice are very much related (see Chapter 13). In the United States, the Dominican Sisters have cared for dying people in the House of Calvary in New York City since 1899. In 1900, another religious order, the Hawthorne Dominicans founded by Rose Hawthorne Lathrope, opened seven homes throughout the country that specialized in the care of dying patients.[1] All of these facilities remain open and functional, although most hospice activities today, as before, provide services through home care programs.

HOME HEALTH SERVICES TODAY

For decades community-based nursing has focused on holistic or total care of the patient and family, as does hospice.[5] This includes response to physical, mental, psychologic, social, cultural, and environmental needs. Home health care agencies continue to expand their services to meet the needs of terminally ill patients. These agencies offer training and in-service programs to improve the skills and abilities of their nurses to provide supportive care at home.

In addition, clinical nursing specialists in oncology and psychiatry are available to many home health agencies on a consulting basis for specific interventions. Physical and occupational therapists, dieticians, and nutritionists also are available for consultation.

The majority of care is provided by nurses, social workers, and home health aides, who represent the basic home care team. Home health aides are analogous to nursing assistants in a hospital. They provide specific treatment under the direction of a nurse, including simple dressings, decubiti care, or assistance with colostomies.

Any patient who expresses a desire to go home and who has supportive family members or friends who are interested, able, and willing to assist, is eligible for home care. In planning for discharge, the patient and family are interviewed and home care needs assessed. Frequently, equipment is ordered for the home, and transportation is arranged for the patient's trip from the hospital. Instruction in management and care is provided to the family or friends before the patient leaves the hospital, and referral to the home care agency is initiated.

The referral includes physician's orders and pertinent information from all health professionals involved in the patient's care, such as nurses, dieticians, social workers, physical therapists, or occupational therapists. The services of physical and occupational therapists, although not necessarily required in the patient's home, are valuable prior to discharge in teaching family members how to move, transfer, and position patients in bed.

Home care services usually begin the day after discharge. The home care nurse visits and thoroughly assesses the patient's physical status, reviews medications and treatments, and checks on any other orders in the plan of care. After discussion with the patient and family, a decision is made about the need for home health aide services. The nurse then communicates with the hospital social work coordinator and hospice nurse coordinator to discuss the plan of care. Volunteer hours are then determined.

Frequent communication among the nurse, palliative care team, and physicians, with occasional joint home visits, usually affords the physical and psychologic support required by the patient and family. Problems generally can be handled without hospital readmission, although in some instances patients are seen in the emergency room and, occasionally, may be readmitted for unexpected difficulties.

A brief case history illustrates the role of home care and the rewarding results of collaborative efforts between the primary physician and the home care nurse.

In addition to his far-advanced lymphoma, Mr. L was totally blind as a result of long-standing diabetes and suffered from hypertension, congestive heart failure, ataxia from a previous stroke, and renal insufficiency. His lymphoma added anemia, weakness, and the need for a Foley catheter for bladder dysfunction to his list of problems. Numerous daily medications were prescribed for his failing organ systems.

When hospital discharge seemed appropriate and the physician initiated discussions toward that goal, Mrs. L, who had cared for her husband's diabetes and other lesser disabilities for many years, protested. She feared that the recent additional complications (especially the care of his catheter) had increased the complexity of home care to the point that she could not handle it, and she insisted on nursing home placement instead. Mr. L refused that option, stating that he would have no reason to continue to live if consigned to a nursing facility. He wanted only to return to his own home.

The discussion was pursued over a period of days with the attending physician, the hospital's discharge-planning nurse, and a visiting nurse representative. They reassured Mrs. L that equipment and assistance would be available to her as needed, and that she could indeed manage to care for her husband at home.

A continuing telephone dialogue was established between the visiting nurse and the physician. This enabled the physician to monitor, by means of the visiting nurse's assessments, the patient's physical status and biochemical parameters (through blood samples drawn by an outpatient laboratory in the patient's home). Dosage adjustments were made as indicated with the nurse providing instructions to the wife. With the help of the visiting nurse and despite her severe apprehensions, Mrs. L coped well, managed ably to maintain her husband at home, and preserved for both of them several months of a much desired and comfortable home-based terminal stage of life.

MEDICARE COVERAGE

The four primary Medicare requirements reflect the conditions and problems that are typical of ongoing home care. First, patients must be homebound and unable to leave the home except for infrequent or brief absences to obtain services in another setting. Second, skilled care must be required for each home visit by a nurse. Observations of a patient per se are not covered, but specific conditions, such as the potential for change in the patient's clinical status, meet the requirement for skilled care. Third, home health aide services must be provided in conjunction with a nurse. Finally, home care services must involve intermittent skilled care for a few hours a day, a few days a week.[3] Occasionally, extended care for up to eight hours a day may be reimbursable when recommended by the physician.

Referral to the home health agency should indicate the need for skilled care, including the need for specific assessment. Assessment includes determination of requirements for skilled care and pain control, and evaluation of cardiovascular, bowel, and bladder status, skin integrity, dietary needs, hydration, and vital signs. Interventions in these areas specifically require a registered nurse, and simultaneously allow for the placement of a home health aide.

Medicare closely scrutinizes the use of home health aides for more than three hours a day over the maximum time allowed, which is four hours a day, five to seven days a week. Volunteers are needed and used to provide assistance in conjunction with home health aides.

Hospitalization of the patient in order to provide a respite for the family is not readily available. To be readmitted, patients typically must have a diagnosis that requires treatment, such as dehydration, malnutrition, infection, or decubitus ulcer. Community hospitals, as opposed to academic medical centers, may be more lenient regarding admission requirements.

In some areas, Medicaid, which is state controlled, will reimburse families that care for the elderly or sick at home. It is an interesting plan which offers incentive to decrease the number of patients requiring long-term institutionalization. It is also a sensible plan; if boarding home owners are paid to care for patients, family members should receive similar reimbursement for their care of relatives in the home. The plan includes the option for admission to a hospital or other facility, such as an extended care facility or skilled nursing home, to enable vacations and rest periods for the family. This service is available and functions well in New York City.

Of course, some patients and/or families cannot or prefer not to manage a death at home. Clearly, home care is neither feasible nor desirable for everyone. The needs of the dying are highly personal and individual. The option to remove care from an impersonal, large institution offers patients the opportunity to maintain their individuality in a familiar environment with their loved ones. Whether our hospice care is provided in the patient's home or in an institution, Saunder's concept encouraging the patient to "live until you die" can be realized.[6]

Through an educational process, health care workers in large institutions can learn to meet the highly variable needs of the dying patient. This degree of individualized attention and concern continues to serve as the basis for home health care.

REFERENCES

1. Waters, Y.: Visiting Nursing in the United States. New York, Charities Publication Committee, 1909.
2. Stewart, J.E.: Home Health Care. St. Louis, C.V. Mosby, 1979.
3. United States General Accounting Office: Hospice Care — A Growing Concept in the U.S. (Report to Congress). Washington, GAO, 1979.
4. Community Health Coordinators Group: Hospital to Home: A Guide to Discharge Planning. Philadelphia, C.D.Q. Printing, 1981.
5. Stoddard, S. (ed.).: The Hospice Movement. New York, Stein and Day, 1978.
6. Saunders, C.: The Management of Terminal Disease. London, Edward Arnold, 1978.

Chapter 13

Hospice

Barrie R.Cassileth
Judy A. Donovan

Hospice is an alternative to standard inpatient care of the dying and is an approach specifically consonant with the needs of the terminally ill. It is an effort to supplement the acute-care model of treatment appropriate to curable stages of disease; it represents an active program of care for patients often treated with inappropriate aggressiveness or simply left to die when death becomes inevitable. The remarkably rapid acceptance and growth of hospice in this country may be attributed to major underlying social changes: new attitudes toward death; biomedical advances that require new understanding of the meaning and definition of death; dissatisfaction with the health care system generally; and an emerging emphasis on the "whole" patient.

THE EVOLUTION OF HOSPICE

Death used to be a forbidden topic. We as a nation avoided the subject, and Ernest Becker's book, *The Denial of Death*, won a Pulitzer Prize for explaining why we did so. We were said to fear the mystery of death and to run from its ugliness, as evidenced by our tendency to die in hospitals rather than at home, and by our expiating, beautifying, expensive funeral rituals. Death was not only an unspoken topic, but a less problematic one as well. Defining death and pinpointing its exact moment in time, for example, became an issue only with the advent of mechanical devices capable of sustaining vital bodily functions despite severe brain injury. Death used to be a certainty, a mystery, a taboo.

No longer. In the last decade, death has entered the public domain—the classroom, the research laboratory, the cocktail party. Depending on one's view, we are compensating for years of silence with a healthy look at a difficult subject or we are morbidly preoccupied with a matter essentially unknowable and best left enigmatic. Regardless, the rise of death and dying to national consciousness and into the spotlight of rational scrutiny is evidenced on many fronts.

School children write poems about death and prepare their epitaphs. The new discipline of thanatology (an ironically euphemistic term for an organized effort to confront and study death openly) has its own journals, conferences, promoters, and professionals. Lay as well as professional publications, films, meetings, and articles abound. College and graduate students can select among a variety of courses focusing on various aspects of death and dying. Experts in law, philosophy, religion, medicine, bioethics, journalism, and education probe and explore this once avoided topic. Death with dignity, facing up to one's personal mortality, letting the patient die, and the like are new and solidly ingrained additions to our vernacular.

The current intense interest in death may be a national effort to capture and dissect a last frontier of human knowledge and experience. It may be perceived also as an attempt to know and prepare for death, and thereby dispel fear. This is a major philosophic and conceptual shift away from the view of death as the grim reaper to one of death as a natural biologic event and, even, "one of the most constructive, positive, and creative elements of culture and life."[1]

Biomedical advances have eradicated most of the infectious illnesses of children and young adults, altering the composition of our population, allowing us to live longer, and vastly increasing the number and proportion of elderly people. This means that more people live to an age when they are increasingly likely to develop chronic diseases such as cancer. Further, it implies that many who do become seriously ill live alone because they are widowed and, therefore, that hospitals and other health care institutions play an expanding custodial, as well as therapeutic, role.

The "biological revolution"[2]—the development of techniques and equipment by which life can be prolonged—changed forever our necessarily passive response to dying and it raised a host of difficult moral, legal, social, and financial issues. Once it became necessary for the public to design living wills and to worry about ensuring permission to die "naturally," death perforce became a pressing social issue. The question of how to handle death and dying thus was foisted upon public consciousness by the facts and implications of the biological revolution.

Another major impetus for the emergence of hospice stemmed from a general dissatisfaction with the American health care system that characterized the past decade. Medicine was curing more diseases and keeping us healthier as a nation, but the American public was dissatisfied as never before. Physical health was only a part of what we desired from our healers. The missing facet, we complained, was a sensitivity to our total selves, a concern on the part of health professionals for the whole patient. Humanistic and holistic medicine became the rallying cry. Appropriate courses, journals, and conferences followed. Books like Illich's *Medical Nemesis* and Carlson's *The End of Medicine*, a new abundance of malpractice suits (20,000 a year and increasing),[3] and a generally anti-medicine and anti-science climate appeared. Hospitals and their lifesaving techniques were castigated for being too institutional, too technologic, and too preoccupied with disease at the expense of the diseased person.

These various interconnected motifs—heightened awareness of death and dying, the biological revolution, dissatisfaction with technologic medicine, and the emphasis on helping the whole person—converged in a new concept of care for the dying: hospice.

HOSPICE CARE

Hospice is a comprehensive program of management that eliminates or de-emphasizes the institutional and technologic aspects of traditional care of the dying. It is interdisciplinary and palliative, focused on symptom relief and psychosocial support for the patient and family when cure or remission is no longer possible. Embodying a commitment to provide all necessary elements of care, hospice management includes pain and other symptom control, emotional and spiritual support, home care when feasible and desired, and bereavement counseling.[4,5] The family, not the patient alone, is the unit of care.

Hospice is not for everyone. However, intrinsic weaknesses in the acute-care hospital's ability to tend to the dying make it a viable option for many. When disease is beyond hope of remission and palliation becomes the treatment goal, hospice broadens the hospital's capacity to provide appropriate and needed care. It offers the physician an additional, vital resource in the continuing effort to provide optimal care. This alternative to aggressive therapy absolutely is not neglect, nor is it a statement of nothing more to offer. Instead, hospice is active intervention aimed specifically at symptom relief and maximum comfort.

Hospice represents a philosophy or program rather than a structure or setting; therefore, it takes many organizational forms. Three approaches predominate, with numerous variations on these basic organizational themes: free-standing hospices; hospital-based programs; and community or home-based hospice programs with no institutional affiliation. One of the first modern hospices, St. Christopher's in England, served as a model for most programs in the United States. Cicely Saunders, a physician, nurse, and social worker, opened St. Christopher's in 1967. The concept spread rapidly throughout England, resulting primarily in the establishment of freestanding units, separate from and independent of hospitals.

Hospice care was initiated in North America less than ten years ago with the opening of the Palliative Care Unit at the Royal Victoria Hospital in Montreal and the Connecticut Hospice in New Haven. By 1981, there were over 800 hospice programs in various stages of development,[6] including 440 operational programs in the United States.

There are relatively few freestanding hospices, or "hospices with walls" in this country; costs associated with maintaining autonomous structures are substantial. Many community-based programs, which serve patients in their homes and are not affiliated with any health care institution exist, particularly in rural areas of the nation. The majority of hospice activities in the United States, however, are hospital-based.

Some hospitals contain separate wards or units for hospice patients in the manner of the Royal Victoria Hospital. Others support a hospice team that provides services to patients wherever they are located in the hospital, and that continues to provide or coordinate care when patients return to their homes. Still other hospital-based programs focus on home care, with inpatient services provided when needed.

Whatever the structure or organization of the hospice program, the multifaceted nature of hospice activity necessitates an interdisciplinary approach. Physicians are involved to varying extents, and typically the patient's primary physician remains closely involved, working in coordination with hospice staff. A combination or subset of social workers, pastoral and other counselors, psychotherapists, physical and occupational therapists, dieticians, and volunteers constitute or serve as consultants to the hospice team. Nurses, however, are the primary caregivers in hospice programs.

Because nurses typically monitor the patient and the therapeutic environment in hospice care, physicians are responsible for sharing their observations with nurses in order to ensure thorough patient assessment. Implicit in this coordination of effort is that nurses are skilled in physical assessment and in accurate interpretation of observed behavior.

The comfort and palliation of terminal patients require constant reassessment of pain, of problems in bowel function, and of nutritional status, followed by appropriate management. Guidelines for managing these and other problems faced by terminal cancer patients are discussed in chapters throughout this book. In hospice, the focus of care at all times is on the patient's comfort. Relief of physical distress is prerequisite to obtaining other kinds of relief, and is best accomplished by the coordinated efforts of physician and nurse.

STANDARDS OF CARE

The National Hospice Organization (NHO) was incorporated in 1978 and by 1980 had become an independent national organization with broad representation. NHO has established guiding principles that have assisted the development of standards in 15 states in which hospice legislation has been instituted or proposed. These principles most likely will continue to guide other states similarly in the future. In addition to their principles, NHO has developed its own standards, which are given below.

THE CURRENT STATUS OF HOSPICE CARE IN THE UNITED STATES

The Joint Commission on Accreditation of Hospitals conducted a national survey of 440 operational hospice programs.[6] It found that 46% of hospice programs are hospital-based, 4% are staffed completely by volunteers, 23% are associated with home health

NATIONAL HOSPICE ORGANIZATION STANDARDS OF HOSPICE CARE[7]

1. The hospice program complies with applicable local, state and federal laws and regulations governing the organization and delivery of health care to patients and families.
2. The hospice program provides a continuum of inpatient and home care services through an integrated administrative structure.
3. The home care services are available 24 hours a day, seven days a week.
4. The patient/family is the unit of care.
5. The hospice program has admission criteria and procedures that reflect: the patient/family's desire and need for service; physician participation; and diagnosis and prognosis.
6. The hospice program seeks to identify, teach, coordinate, and supervise persons to give care to patients who do not have a family member available.
7. The hospice program acknowledges that each patient/family has its own beliefs and/or value system and is respectful of them.
8. Hospice care consists of a blending of professional and nonprofessional services, provided by an interdisciplinary team, including a medical director.
9. Staff support is an integral part of the hospice program.
10. Inservice training and continuing education are offered on a regular basis.
11. The goal of hospice care is to provide symptom control through appropriate palliative therapies.
12. Symptom control includes assessing and responding to the physical, emotional, social, and spiritual needs of the patient/family.
13. The hospice program provides bereavement services to survivors for a period of at least one year.
14. There will be a quality assurance program that includes evaluation of services, regular chart audits, and organizational review.
15. The hospice program maintains accurate and current integrated records on all patient/families.
16. The hospice complies with all applicable state and federal regulations.
17. The hospice inpatient unit provides space for patient/family privacy, visitation, and viewing, and for food preparation by the family.

agencies, and 26% combine case manager, visiting nurse association, and community-based home care.

Cancer patients constitute the vast majority of hospice patients, and hospice programs now serve 25 to 40% of dying cancer patients in their service areas.[8] The typical hospice patient seeks or is referred to hospice care having been treated unsuccessfully in traditional health care settings. Most patients enter hospice programs with chronic, unrelieved pain and unmanaged, severe emotional and spiritual stress. It is precisely these problems that hospice endeavors to correct.

An actuarial study indicates that costs associated with hospice care generally are substantially lower than costs of traditional treatment during terminal illness.[9] By eliminating expensive diagnostic and therapeutic measures when they are not indicated, by focusing on home care when appropriate and feasible, and by primarily emphasizing nursing rather than physician involvement, hospice offers substantial cost savings while simultaneously providing services that are more in keeping with the dying person's clinical and psychosocial needs.[10-12] These savings are feasible because hospice is an alternative, not an addition, to traditional care of the terminally ill.

Acceptance of hospice is evidenced by the speed with which numerous programs have evolved, by substantial accrual to these programs, by frequent and positive media coverage, and by private and public financial support.[13] Although the humanitarian and clinical goals of hospice—minimizing the physical and spiritual pain of terminal illness—have been accepted broadly, the future direction of hospice is unclear. Federal policy and reimbursement mechanisms will determine in large part if and how hospice goals will be implemented and positioned in the health care system.

ACCREDITATION AND REIMBURSEMENT

It is generally agreed that accreditation and licensure will bring hospice more solidly into the health care system and will facilitate third-party reimbursement. However, which organization is best suited to grant accreditation remains undetermined. Several existing health and government agencies would like to control or participate in accreditation policies. Some states have their own accreditation programs. The issue of national versus state accreditation is as yet unresolved, with good arguments for each possibility.

Whatever accreditation or licensing mechanisms emerge in the future, the question of reimbursement will not automatically be addressed. Reimbursement remains one of the most important and difficult problems of the hospice movement. A bill introduced to the United States Congress in December, 1981, deals in part with the reimbursement issue. The bill would amend the Social Security Act to provide hospice benefits, as part of hospital insurance coverage, to people eligible for Medicare benefits. Nationally, approximately 70% of hospice patients are eligible for Medicare and thus would receive the hospice benefit.

The proposed hospice coverage would allow Medicare beneficiaries who are considered by their physicians to have less than six months to live to receive services from a bona fide hospice program. This would involve no additional cost to the Medicare trust fund. Instead, hospice care would be substituted for more expensive acute care, with substantial savings to the Medicare system.[14]

Until this bill is enacted, or until third-party payors on more than a demonstration basis recognize hospice for its unique, comprehensive and cost-efficient services, most hospice programs will continue to provide care without direct reimbursement. It would be unfortunate if, as anticipated, many hospice programs prove unable to survive under present reimbursement regulations.

If that occurs, hospice will cease to be an available option. We will be forced to continue providing unnecessarily expensive services in the traditional hospital setting, an environment ill-prepared to deliver the character of care that many terminally ill patients and their physicians want and require.

REFERENCES

1. Kubler-Ross, E.: Death: The Final Stage of Growth. Prentice-Hall, Englewood Cliffs, New Jersey, 1975.
2. Veatch, R.M.: Death, Dying, and the Biological Revolution: Our Last Quest for Responsibility. New Haven, Yale University Press, 1976.
3. Newsweek magazine: June 9, p. 59, 1976.
4. Lack, S.A.: Hospice—a concept of care in the final stages of life. Conn. Med., *43*:367–372, 1979.
5. Zimmerman, J.M.: Hospice—Complete Care for the Terminally Ill. Baltimore, Urban and Schwarzenberg, 1981.
6. JCAH: Interim Report on Hospice. Chicago, JCAH, July, 1981.
7. NHO Standards of Hospice Care, National Hospice Organization, 301 Maple Avenue West, Vienna, VA 22180, Nov., 1981.
8. Gaetz, D.: The case for hospice from a hospital persepective. Am. Protestant Hosp. Assoc. Bull. *45*:33–40, 1981.
9. Fullerton, W.D., Wolkstein, I., Hash, M.M., and Zwick, D.I.: Cost Analysis of Proposed Hospice Reimbursement Bill. Commissioned by the Warner-Lambert Foundation. Health Policy Alternatives, Inc., 545 8th St. SE, Washington, D.C., Nov., 1981.
10. Zimmerman, J.M.: Experience with a hospice-care program for the terminally ill. Ann. Surg., *189*:683–690, 1979.
11. Bloom, B.S., and Kissick, P.D.: Home and hospital cost of terminal illness. Med. Care, *18*:560–564, 1980.
12. U.S. General Accounting Office: Hospice Care: A Growing Concept in the United States. HRD-79-50 (March 6, 1979).
13. Martin, M.C.: Hospice care update: many questions still to be answered. Hospitals, *55*:56–59, 1981.

14. U.S., Congress, House: A bill to Amend Title XVIII of the Social Security Act to Provide for Coverage of Hospice Care under the Medicare Program. H.R. 5180, 97th Cong., 1st session, 1981.

Chapter 14

Legal and Ethical Issues

Arnold Rosoff

The dilemma of when to discontinue treatment of terminally ill patients has received wide exposure in the media. Almost daily we see references to court proceedings seeking legal authorization to terminate therapy for individuals in irreversible coma or facing imminent death. Clinicians, it seems, are extremely apprehensive about the legal implications of these difficult life-or-death decisions. Based on earlier court decisions, much of this concern is deserved. On the other hand, in recent years the law has become more sensitive to these medico-legal issues and to the pressures upon professionals working in this emotionally charged area of health care. The law on this subject is in flux, with frequent additions both to statutory and case law. Providers of care to the terminally ill should stay abreast of these developments. It is to this end that the present chapter is addressed.

THE LEGAL BACKGROUND

Before turning to the specific issue of terminal care, we should consider briefly some general principles of medical jurisprudence and the evolving doctrine of "informed consent." When we speak of "law," we are talking essentially about duties and rights: the *duty* of an individual to do, or refrain from doing, something and the *right* of the other party to have it done or not done. The duties here are those of the provider of health care and the corresponding rights belong to the patient. Basically, the patients' rights are the following: to be treated with due care and not to be treated against

their will. Identifying the sources of the provider's duty will help
in evaluating its nature and extent.

Contract Law

In the medical care context, the provider's duty to the patient
falls basically under one of two major categories of the law, contract
and tort. The Latin legal term for contract, "assumpsit," is instructive. It means "he assumed," or "he undertook." When physicians undertake to treat a patient, they make a commitment to
the patient to render the agreed upon care consistent with generally accepted professional standards.

In contract litigation, the primary inquiry often is to ascertain
the intent of the parties, in other words, "What is it that the party
in question undertook to do?" The terms of a commercial contract
typically are spelled out in detail. In the medical context, however,
the nature of the physician-patient relationship and the state of
the patient's health often preclude explicit advance articulation of
what is to be done. During the course of treatment, particularly
with terminally ill patients, the understanding between patient
and physician can change with the patient's condition. It becomes
difficult, then, to identify at a given time what the implicit terms
of the relationship are.

Whenever people present themselves for care and the clinician
undertakes to provide that care, an implied contract comes into
being. In attempting to identify its terms and unspoken understandings, the law looks to the general practice of the medical
profession, subject, of course, to any contrary understandings that
the provider and patient may have reached. This reference to
professional standards is essentially the same approach that is used
to define performance standards for tort law purposes.

Tort Law

The second main source of the physician's legal duty is tort
law. A "tort" is a civil wrong: an injury done to person, property,
or reputation. In medicine, the relevant element is injury to one's
person, the physical body. Whereas a contractual relationship is
not created unless one voluntarily undertakes an obligation, all of

us by virtue of living in society are obliged not to act in a way that harms others.

Although some torts are deliberate, most result from negligence. As defined by our legal system, negligence is predicated upon four elements, often termed "the four D's." The first is *Duty*. In order to hold someone liable for a negligent tort, one must first establish that the actor owed a duty of care and what that duty was. Second, one must show *Dereliction* of that duty, that the individual fell significantly short of the standard of reasonably expected care. Third, *Damage* to the complainant must be proven. The fourth element is *Direct Causation*, namely, the damage must be shown to have been caused *directly* by the dereliction of duty. The negligence cannot be simply a contributing factor toward the harm suffered; it must be the "proximate cause," without which the damage would not have occurred.

In tort law, the duty of care generally is measured by reference to the tort-feasor's peers. Dereliction is a matter of judgment for jury or judge. The question is whether the defendant physician deviated significantly from the requisite standard of care. In the health care context, duty commonly is based upon norms within the medical profession. The standard of care is defined in terms of what a hypothetical "reasonable, prudent practitioner" would do under the same or similar circumstances, a matter of fact that usually must be established by expert medical testimony.

Estoppel

In addition to tort and contract law, yet another basis exists upon which the clinician's obligations may be grounded. When a doctor and patient enter into a relationship, the patient develops certain reasonable expectations about what will be done. Unilateral frustration of those expectations by the physician is actionable. "Estoppel" is the legal term for the concept that one who causes another to rely in a foreseeable way is obliged to act so as not to frustrate that reliance. For example, suppose a patient submits to care believing that the physician will do everything reasonably feasible to sustain life. Should the physician independently determine that the patient is too far gone to attempt to sustain or resuscitate life, it could be argued that the physician is bound nonetheless by estoppel to render the care expected by the patient.

Alternatively, it could be reasoned that the provision of such care is an implied term of the physician-patient contract. Variance between what one person expects to get and what the other gives—a difference between the expectations on one side and the commitment on the other—creates the potential for legal liability. Such cases may be treated as raising issues of estoppel or of contract; the two principles are closely related when they arise in this context.

It often happens that patients fail to express in advance their wishes regarding treatment in the terminal stage. Acting with humane intent, the physician may issue a "No code" or "Do not resuscitate" order. If family members learn of this, they could claim that the physician violated the implicit terms of the treatment contract. "We thought that you were going to do everything you could to save our relative," they might complain. The legal question thus raised would be, in refraining from a resuscitation attempt, did the physician act as other responsible medical professionals would have in the same situation? Even if there were, in fact, a frustration of the patient's unstated expectations, liability would not likely be found if the defendant proved that resuscitation at this stage is not common and that the physician's action, therefore, was consistent with commonly accepted medical judgment and practice.

INFORMED CONSENT

A related issue is that of consent, a concept that evolved from the tort law of assault and/or battery. A "battery" is an unpermitted touching of someone and includes even the most minimal invasion of bodily privacy. If someone were to touch another without permission, even if it was an inoffensive, friendly pat on the back, technically that would be a battery. "Assault" means placing someone in fear of a battery. One who lunges out and stops just short of hitting another's nose has committed assault, but has not committed a battery. On the other hand, an unconscious person can be battered in the absence of assault. Judge Cardozo, later a U.S. Supreme Court Justice, stated a principle in the 1914 New York case, *Schloendorff* v. *Society of New York Hospital*, which has come to be regarded as the "root premise" in the law of consent to health care. He said, "Every human being of adult years and sound mind has a right to determine what is to be done with his own body, and a physician who undertakes an operation without the patient's consent commits an assault, for which he is liable in damages."[1]

From the turn of the century through the 1950s, questions of consent were rather simple "yes-or-no" matters. If there was a signed consent document, or if someone could establish that the patient had given oral consent, the law was satisfied. The patient's thought process and degree of understanding were not questioned. All that mattered was whether formal consent had been given.

The consent issue changed in 1957 with the case of *Salgo* v. *Stanford University Board of Trustees*.[2] A patient had signed a consent form for an aortogram. The rare occurrence of paralysis from the procedure had not been explained to her. When paralysis occurred, she claimed that she had not meaningfully consented to the procedure. The consent form was introduced as evidence by the defendants. The plaintiff argued that consent given in the absence of knowledge and understanding is without legal effect. The court agreed, holding that unless consent is educated, or "informed," even if formally correct, it is legally inadequate. The *Salgo* case did not specify what information should be disclosed to the patient. It simply recognized that the validity of consent depends on the patient's adequate understanding of the authorized procedure.

An important court decision three years later further confirmed the point that a patient's consent must be informed to be legally effective. In *Natanson* v. *Kline* (1960), the Kansas Supreme Court held that what a physician must disclose in order to obtain "informed consent" should be measured by standards traditionally applied in negligence cases, namely, those of the relevant professional community.[3] The standard of disclosure, then, is what a reasonable, prudent practitioner commonly would disclose in the same or similar circumstances. This measure, the court felt, was as applicable to questions of information disclosure as to questions of how particular surgical procedures should be performed. Obviously, the court believed that it was possible, as a factual matter, to discern a professional consensus on revelation of treatment information.

From a legal perspective, something interesting happened in *Natanson:* two branches of tort law were combined. The court took the basic notion of consent from battery law and made it operational by using a principle from negligence law. The result was greater autonomy for the medical profession, because its obligation of disclosure was tied to professional practice rather than to patients' needs or desires for information.

Throughout the 1960s, informed consent cases arose in ever larger numbers as the consumer movement flourished generally in this country. The viability of those suits was seriously compromised, however, by application of negligence law principles, as per *Natanson*. Patient-plaintiffs wishing to complain that their consent was uninformed had to locate medical witnesses willing to testify as to what the "average, prudent practitioner" would have disclosed. Then they had to show that the defendant-physician had revealed significantly less, had misrepresented, or had concealed information normally a part of such "standard disclosure." If the patient could not find expert witnesses to testify that doctors typically disclose such information, the patient had no case sufficient to go to a jury. The reluctance of physicians to testify against their peers undoubtedly kept many consent cases from being prosecuted successfully. Moreover, even if witnesses could be found, this would not help the plaintiff if the professional consensus was to limit disclosure. Medical practitioners could join hands, in effect, by regularly providing minimal explanations to patients, thus lowering the legal standard by which all physicians' disclosures would be measured.

A significant case undercut this physician-based standard and substantially altered the law of consent. That case was *Canterbury* v. *Spence*,[4] decided in 1972 by the U.S. Court of Appeals for the District of Columbia Circuit. The *Canterbury* case involved a 19-year-old man who underwent a laminectomy by a neurosurgeon without being advised in advance of any risks or possible side effects of the operation. The patient became partially paralyzed following the operation and sued, charging the physician with negligence in performing the surgery and with failing to obtain an adequately "informed" consent. At trial, the defendant neurosurgeon admitted that there is a risk of paralysis inherent in any laminectomy, a risk that he reckoned to approximate one per cent. The patient's attorney asked Dr. Spence why he had not informed his patient of this risk. The doctor responded that disclosure would have been medically unwise:

> I think that I always explain to patients the operations are serious, and I feel that any operation is serious. I think that I would not tell patients that they might be paralyzed because of the small percentage, one per cent, that exists. There would be a tremendous percentage of people that would

not have surgery and would not therefore be benefited by it, the tremendous percentage that get along very well, 99 per cent.[5]

The physician, in effect, was saying that he does not tell patients about risks associated with laminectomy in order to avoid the possibility that some patients would decide contrary to his judgment. The court did not take kindly to this paternalistic approach and was prompted to establish a new rule based on enhanced respect for the principle of individual self-determination. The *Canterbury* case substantially altered the doctrine of informed consent by replacing the medical-professional standard of acceptable action with a patient-based standard. Said the court:

> . . .We do not agree that the patient's cause of action is dependent upon the existence and nonperformance of a relevant professional tradition.
>
> There are, in our view, formidable obstacles to acceptance of the notion that the physician's obligation to disclose is either germinated or limited by medical practice. To begin with, the reality of any discernible custom reflecting a professional consensus on communication of option and risk information to patients is open to serious doubt. We sense the danger that what in fact is no custom at all may be taken as an affirmative custom to maintain silence, and that physician-witnesses to the so-called custom may state merely their personal opinions as to what they or others would do under given conditions. Nor can we ignore the fact that to bind the disclosure obligation to medical usage is to arrogate the decision on revelation to the physician alone. Respect for the patient's right of self-determination on particular therapy demands a standard set by law for physicians rather than one which physicians may or may not impose upon themselves.[6]

The point of this quote is clear: the law does not believe that applying a physician-based disclosure standard adequately protects the patient's right of self-determination. Operationally, the *Canterbury* case shifted the duty of disclosure from what doctors commonly reveal and made it turn, instead, upon what patients commonly would want to know. What must be divulged is everything that an average, reasonable patient, under similar circumstances, would consider material to the decision whether to authorize the therapy. This includes information regarding the diagnosis; the nature and purpose of the proposed treatment; the risks and likely consequences of that treatment; the probability that the treatment will be successful; reasonably feasible treatment alternatives; and the prognosis if no treatment is given. With regard to risks, the necessity of disclosure is basically a function of the probability of the harmful outcome multiplied by the severity of the harm.

Philosophically, this shift from a doctor-based to a patient-based disclosure standard is most significant. In practice it is even more important, for it frees potential plaintiffs from the need to secure expert testimony on the "slippery" question of what physicians normally disclose to patients. With this evidentiary obstacle reduced, patients can institute "informed consent" suits far more readily. This is precisely the impact reflected in medical malpractice litigation statistics since 1972. The issue of "informed consent" has assumed a much more prominent place in the consciousness of and the law suits against health care providers.

The new standard enunciated in the *Canterbury* case has been adopted by roughly half of the states. The rest still hold to the old doctor-based rule. In all states, however, physicians should assume that the law strongly supports patients' rights to be informed about their condition, the therapy proposed, treatment alternatives, and the prognosis if no treatment is given. Elaborate detail is not required; a simple, understandable explanation in lay terms is preferable to a complex, technical disquisition. Neither remote possibilities nor matters of common knowledge need be disclosed. Further, the duty of disclosure is subject to two exceptions. No disclosure is required if the patient indicates a preference not to be informed or if the provider believes, in the exercise of sound medical judgment, that the patient is so anxiety-prone or disturbed that the information would not be processed rationally or that it would probably cause significant psychologic harm. The latter exception to the duty of disclosure often is referred to as "therapeutic privilege" and is recognized in most jurisdictions, although the courts are careful to limit its application so that the basic disclosure obligation is not unduly undermined. The *Canterbury* court stated well this limitation in responding to Dr. Spence's testimony that he commonly withheld information to keep his patients from making the "wrong" decisions on therapy:

> The physician's privilege to withhold information for therapeutic reasons must be carefully circumscribed, however, for otherwise it might devour the disclosure rule itself. The privilege does not accept the paternalistic notion that the physician may remain silent simply because divulgence might prompt the patient to forego therapy the physician feels the patient really needs.[7]

Thus, when the provider withholds information under either of the above exceptions, the facts supporting this decision should be carefully documented. As to the latter exception, consultation with another physician familiar with the patient, with a close associate of the patient, or both, can help to supply the needed documentation.

CARE OF THE DYING PATIENT

With the basic principles of "informed consent" as background, we can consider their application to the terminally ill patient. Because the law so scrupulously guards patients' rights to decide on their own care, one might assume that patients are free also to reject care intended to prolong a life that is rapidly passing. Unfortunately, at least insofar as a simple answer is desired, the law is not that clear. Courts have held that a person does not have a legally protected "right to die." Suicide is still a crime in many states. On occasion, patients' refusals of blood transfusions and other life-saving procedures have been overridden by court orders authorizing health care providers to administer needed therapy. However, virtually all of these cases have involved situations in which recovery to normal functioning could be expected if the procedure in question were performed. Courts have not interfered with the choice of competent adult patients to refuse "heroic" or artificial life-support measures when death was imminent. No case law suggests that in such extreme situations the decision of a rational patient should not be respected, or that a physician would be liable for following the patient's wishes by withholding or discontinuing extraordinary life-support measures.

As is true of consent generally, it is extremely important to document that the termination of care or the exclusive application of palliative care does, in fact, reflect the patient's wishes and that the patient is competent to make such a choice. The so-called "Living Will," even though its use may not be legislatively approved in a given jurisdiction, provides such documentation. The standard form of a Living Will speaks to situations in which patients are unable to express their wishes any longer because of coma or other inability to communicate (Fig. 14–1). However, a variant of this document can be devised for use while the patient is still fully competent and able to communicate. Such a document records the patient's wish that only palliative care should be given once the physician has determined that further curative therapy would be unavailing. A sample document for this purpose is provided in Figure 14–2.

This informed consent document is direct in its approach to a sensitive subject. As compared with the more general language of the "Living Will," which often is signed when a person is not *in extremis*, it might seem blunt in its reference to the lack of hope

To My Family, My Physician, My Lawyer and All Others Whom It May Concern

Death is as much a reality as birth, growth, maturity and old age—it is the one certainty of life. If the time comes when I can no longer take part in decisions for my own future, let this statement stand as an expression of my wishes and directions, while I am still of sound mind.

If at such a time the situation should arise in which there is no reasonable expectation of my recovery from extreme physical or mental disability, I direct that I be allowed to die and not be kept alive by medications, artificial means or "heroic measures". I do, however, ask that medication be mercifully administered to me to alleviate suffering even though this may shorten my remaining life.

This statement is made after careful consideration and is in accordance with my strong convictions and beliefs. I want the wishes and directions here expressed carried out to the extent permitted by law. Insofar as they are not legally enforceable, I hope that those to whom this Will is addressed will regard themselves as morally bound by these provisions.

Signed _____

Date _____

Witness _____

Witness _____

Copies of this request have been given to _____

_____

_____

_____

Fig. 14–1. A Living Will.

IMPORTANT

Declarants may wish to add specific statements to the Living Will to be inserted in the space provided for that purpose above the signature. Possible additional provisions are suggested below:

1. a) I appoint _____
   to make binding decisions concerning my medical treatment.

   OR

   b) I have discussed my views as to life sustaining measures with the following who understand my wishes

   _____,
   _____,
   _____.

2. Measures of artificial life support in the face of impending death that are especially abhorrent to me are:
   a) Electrical or mechanical resuscitation of my heart when it has stopped beating.
   b) Nasogastric tube feedings when I am paralyzed and no longer able to swallow.
   c) Mechanical respiration by machine when my brain can no longer sustain my own breathing.
   d) _____

3. If it does not jeopardize the chance of my recovery to a meaningful and sentient life or impose an undue burden on my family, I would like to live out my last days at home rather than in a hospital.

4. If any of my tissues are sound and would be of value as transplants to help other people, I freely give my permission for such donation.

**INFORMED CONSENT
TO PROVISION OF ONLY PALLIATIVE CARE
IN THE TREATMENT OF TERMINAL ILLNESS**

I have been informed that I am suffering from_____
[INSERT DESCRIPTION OF PATIENT'S DISEASE]

_____

_____

and that further attempts to achieve a cure or attain a significant remission are not likely to be successful. All of my questions concerning this determination have been answered to my full satisfaction by [NAME OF ATTENDING PHYSI-CIAN]. It is my carefully considered decision that further care rendered to me should be limited to palliative measures appropriate to assuring my physical and emotional comfort and the preservation of my personal dignity. If necessary to relieve terminal suffering, I request that pain-suppressing drugs be administered to me even though this may hasten my death.

    With full realization of what I am asking, I sincerely request that any person(s) having responsibility for my care will respect my wishes recorded herein and that any person so doing will be held harmless from any legal liability in connection therewith.

DATE: _____   SIGNED:_____
                                                            (PATIENT'S NAME)

WITNESS: _____

       (NEXT OF KIN, IF AVAILABLE)

Fig. 14–2. Document recording patient's wish to receive only palliative care once the physician determines that cure is impossible.

for recovery. Long-standing medical tradition appears to favor the use of equivocal statements and euphemisms to sustain hope as long as possible. From a legal standpoint, however, directness and honesty are not only favored, they are essential to legally effective consent. Thus, if a provider were to decide unilaterally that a particular patient's condition merited no further attempts at cure and thereafter rendered only palliative care, this approach would be actionable if it were inconsistent with the patient's knowledge-able decision. Even the involvement and concurrence of the patient's close relatives would not legitimate a decision made without consultation with a competent, adult patient. Dealing directly with the patient, therefore, is generally the best course to follow. A reasonable, sound protection against a potential lawsuit is to have the patient execute a document of the type just proposed.

CASE LAW ON THE "RIGHT TO DIE"

The preceding recommendations are based upon analysis of recent court decisions concerning termination of treatment. Although case law increasingly reflects a judicial tendency to accept patients' decisions on termination, one must recognize that the relevant legal principles are not yet definitively established. Moreover, the law may vary considerably from state to state; a prominent decision in one state, although it may be highly persuasive in others, is not binding on the courts of other states. Thus the principles discussed in the following pages, except in the particular states from which they are drawn, are merely educated inferences as to how other states would decide in similar situations.

The Quinlan Case

Probably every physician knows at least the basic facts of the *Karen Quinlan* case.[8] In this precedent-setting 1976 decision, the Supreme Court of New Jersey held that it was legally acceptable to withdraw artificial life-support measures from a comatose patient who had suffered severe, irreversible brain damage and who could not reasonably be expected ever to return to a "cognitive, sapient state." In reaching that decision, the court relied heavily upon the constitutionally protected "right of privacy" articulated by the United States Supreme Court in *Roe* v. *Wade*,[9] the controversial 1973 decision recognizing a woman's right to abortion. The right to make decisions about one's own health care, the High Court held in *Wade*, may be contravened by the state only when there is a "compelling state interest." The *Quinlan* court found the state to have no such compelling interest in a person who could not be expected ever to regain meaningful consciousness. It then articulated the following calculus for determining when the state is exceeding its limits in maintaining a person's life by extraordinary means:

> . . . We think that the State's interest *contra* weakens and the individual's right to privacy grows as the degree of bodily invasion increases and the prognosis dims. Ultimately there comes a point at which the individual's rights overcome the State interest. . . [10]

Having established the basic right of a patient to elect termination of life-support measures, the court went on to hold that Karen's adoptive father, Joseph Quinlan, could make that decision on her behalf, guided by a good faith belief as to what the patient would choose for herself if able to formulate and express her decision. This concept of "substituted judgment," although the *Quinlan* court did not so label it, has become firmly embedded in the law on termination of care.

An important procedural point about the *Quinlan* case is that the court did not intend judicial intervention to be a regular requirement in termination of care cases. Instead, the court felt that such matters should be left to a patient's legal guardian and attending physicians, but with obligatory involvement of the hospital's ethics committee for the limited purpose of confirming the physicians' prognosis that a return to cognitive life could not reasonably be expected. Thus, the court attempted to regularize these decisions by providing an extrajudicial process that respects the pressures of clinical decision-making while still providing a measure of safety against hasty or improperly motivated action. Such reliance upon hospital committees has been approved by other courts and by some legislative enactments as well.

The Religious View and "Extraordinary Care"

Of interest and importance is the fact that no major western religious group objected to the decision in the *Quinlan* case. In fact, Joseph Quinlan, a devoted Catholic, was supported by his church in requesting termination of artificial life support for his daughter. As early as 1957, Pope Pius XII declared that prolonging the dying process by extraordinary medical measures was not required. In so saying, the Pontiff echoed the prevalent clerical view that artificial maintenance of bodily functions *in extremis* interferes with the natural process of death and is not supportable in the absence of hope for recovery. The Pope also recognized the complex psychosocial aspects of terminal illness when he observed that not only the needs of the patient, but also the economic and emotional impact of prolonged dying upon the family and attending staff should be considered in such cases.[11]

Of course, the question remains of how to define "extraordinary care." Certainly, many medical techniques and devices taken for granted today would have seemed extraordinary a few years ago. Technologic advance renders "standard practice" a moving target. However, the Papal pronouncement again provides guidance, by defining as "extraordinary," care "which cannot be obtained or used without excessive expense, pain, or other inconvenience, or which, if used, would not offer a reasonable hope of benefit."[12] Most courts today would support such a definition.

The Saikewicz Case

In 1977, the Supreme Judicial Court of Massachusetts decided *Superintendent of Belchertown State School* v. *Saikewicz*,[13] a case that received almost as much attention in the medical press as *Quinlan*. Following essentially the principles established by the *Quinlan* court, the Massachusetts high court held that it was legally acceptable for the guardian of an incompetent ward of the state to reject on the ward's behalf a chemotherapeutic regimen to treat leukemia. The patient, Joseph Saikewicz, was a 67-year-old man with a mental age of 3 who had been institutionalized for most of his life. Because the patient could not decide for himself whether to undergo chemotherapy, the concept of "substituted judgment" again was invoked. The question posed to the court was, "What would the patient choose for himself if he had the ability to do so?" Here a special problem was encountered, in that the court acknowledged that most people in their sixties probably would elect therapy, even if the chances of success were minimal. The key difference, the court observed, was that Saikewicz would not be able to comprehend the purpose of the treatment and, thus, probably would find it far less tolerable than would an individual who could understand what was happening to him. Beginning with a quote from the incompetent's guardian *ad litem*, the court reasoned:

> . . ."If he is treated with toxic drugs he will be involuntarily immersed in a state of painful suffering, the reason for which he will never understand. Patients who request treatment know the risks involved and can appreciate the painful side-effects when they arrive. They know the reason for the pain and their hope makes it tolerable." To make a worthwhile comparison, one would have to ask whether a majority of people would choose chemotherapy if they were told merely that something outside of their previous experience was going to be done to them, that this something would cause them pain and discomfort, that they would be removed to strange surroundings and possibly restrained for extended periods of time, and that the advantages of this course of action were measured by concepts of time and mortality beyond their ability to comprehend.[14]

"Substituted judgment," *Saikewicz* thus holds, must be applied with regard for the special circumstances of the particular patient. The question is not what the "average, reasonable patient" would desire, although this information may be instructive. Rather, it is what this particular patient would want, insofar as this can be deduced by others who genuinely have the patient's best interest at heart.

Medical professionals, while accepting of the court's substantive decision in *Saikewicz*, were nevertheless greatly distressed by the procedure that the court announced it would require in such cases, to wit, regular submission to judicial determination. Said the court:

> . . .We take a dim view of any attempt to shift the ultimate decision-making responsibility away from the duly established courts of proper jurisdiction to any committee, panel or group, ad hoc or permanent. Thus, we reject the approach adopted by the New Jersey Supreme Court in the *Quinlan* case of entrusting the decision whether to continue artificial life support to the patient's guardian, family, attending doctors, and hospital "ethics committee.". . .
>
> We do not view the judicial resolution of this most difficult and awesome question—whether potentially life-prolonging treatment should be withheld from a person incapable of making his own decision—as constituting a "gratuitous encroachment" on the domain of medical expertise. Rather, such questions of life and death seem to us to require the process of detached but passionate investigation and decision that forms the ideal on which the judicial branch was created. Achieving this ideal is our responsibility and that of the lower court, and is not to be entrusted to any other group purporting to represent the "morality and conscience of our society," no matter how highly motivated or impressively constituted.[15]

The need for regular resort to the courts in such situations, which seemed impossibly burdensome to the New Jersey court, thus was accepted in Massachusetts, or so it seemed at the time. Later cases, including *In Re Dinnerstein*, which will be discussed shortly, have made it clear that Massachusetts will not require all termination of treatment cases to be brought before its courts.

The Case of Brother Fox

The aforementioned recommendation that the patient's wish to receive only palliative care be documented is supported by a recent, much publicized decision of the New York courts. In *Application of Father Phillip K. Eichner, S.M.*,[16] the New York Court of Appeals, the state's highest court, held that there is a common law right to refuse artificial life-support and that this right survives the incompetency of an individual if "clear and convincing evidence" exists that the patient elected such refusal while of sound mind. The patient in this case, Brother Fox, an 83-year-old member of the Society of Mary, had often and publicly expressed his belief in Pope Pius XII's pronouncements on artificial life support and his desire not to be maintained by "extraordinary means" if ever in a condition like that of Karen Quinlan. When such an unfortunate circumstance did arise, his religious superior, Father Eichner, petitioned the New York court to have Brother Fox removed from the respirator that maintained him in a permanent, vegetative state. A key factor in the court's decision to withdraw such support was clear proof of Brother Fox's wishes on this precise point. Still, consistent with the *Saikewicz* holding in Massachusetts, the New York court declared that judicial intervention is required before life support can be withdrawn.

LEGISLATIVE SOLUTIONS: "NATURAL DEATH" ACTS

The cases just described are only a sampling of the voluminous judicial activity of the past several years dealing with the termination of treatment issue. However, the myriad of specific contexts in which this issue arises makes the slow, case-by-case development of legal principles a poor solution to the dilemma that physicians routinely face in treating terminally ill patients.

The so-called "Natural Death" acts, adopted by several states since the *Quinlan* case drew national attention to this issue in 1976, provide some guidance. The statutes enacted by various state legislatures leave much to be desired both in the completeness of their coverage and in the wisdom of the procedures they establish. Nonetheless, they are a welcome first step toward securing the individual rights of the terminally ill and protecting the practitioners who care for them. A brief introduction to these laws and to the procedures they authorize follows.

The first Natural Death act was adopted in California,[17,18] about half a year after the *Quinlan* decision. This law proclaims the right of an adult, "qualified patient" to execute a "directive" that life-sustaining procedures should be withheld or withdrawn in the event of a terminal condition. Written diagnosis and certification of the terminal condition are required from two physicians to establish that a patient is "qualified." The directive is not fully effective until 14 days have elapsed *after* such certification. This waiting period is imposed to guard against the possibility that patients may act out of despair immediately after learning that their condition is terminal. A properly executed directive imposes a duty upon the physician to refrain from life-sustaining procedures:

> which, when applied to a qualified patient, would serve only to artificially prolong the moment of death and where, in the judgment of the attending physician, death is imminent whether or not such procedures are utilized. "Life-sustaining procedure" shall not include the administration of medication or the performance of any medical procedure deemed necessary to alleviate pain.[19]

A physician who complies with a properly executed directive is shielded from civil or criminal liability for so doing. On the other hand, physicians who do not wish to comply with such a directive are not compelled to do so, but they must transfer the care of the patient to another physician willing to execute the directive. Failure to effect such a transfer is deemed "unprofessional conduct."

Note that the California law applies only to cases in which death is "imminent," whether or not life-sustaining treatment is provided. Thus, it does not recognize a "right to die," but merely a right not to have the process of death unduly prolonged. The word "imminent" is not defined in the statute, but is generally understood in a clinical setting to mean that death can be expected to occur within a few hours or, at most, a few days. Although greater specificity might seem desirable, it probably would make little difference in practice, because it is rarely possible to predict precisely the moment of death.

California's statute, despite its considerable detail, has significant omissions. It neglects the subject of minors or incompetents as well as the situation in which a person is stricken suddenly, as in an automobile accident, and thus has no chance to execute a directive. The statute covers, then, only a small segment of the overall spectrum of "termination of treatment" situations.

The flurry of legislation that followed the *Quinlan* case has substantially abated. New and difficult cases, as they arise from time to time, will rekindle interest in this type of legislation. Statutory law dealing with at least some aspects of the termination of treatment issue probably will be adopted in all states. Practitioners should check periodically with relevant state sources, such as the department of health, the attorney general's office, and medical societies, to learn about statute-and-case law that guides and constrains decisions in this difficult area.

ORDERS NOT TO RESUSCITATE

There comes a time in the care of most terminally ill patients when a decision must be made regarding attempts to resuscitate in the event of cardiac or pulmonary arrest. Ideally, this decision would be made in consultation with the patient, whose wishes should be recorded and respected. As a practical matter, however, the issue often arises when the patient is too debilitated to participate in the decision or when the physician feels that confronting the patient with the issue of death would be inhumane. At this point, a "rule of reason" should be applied. Even though patients theoretically may be entitled to decide for themselves, it is highly unlikely that a court would hold liable physicians who follow their conscience in not insisting upon the exercise of that "right." Note, however, that this observation applies only in a case in which the patient's condition is clearly terminal.

Commonly, when the attending physician determines that resuscitation should not be attempted, this decision is discussed with the patient's next of kin or other close relatives. Oral communication is usually all that is involved, although the physician would be well advised to secure a written "release" from family members present if the existence of consensus is in any doubt. Nevertheless, relatives of the patient, even the next of kin, have no power to authorize termination of treatment. However, their recorded concurrence in this decision, assuming the patient's condition was fully and accurately revealed to them, will estop them from later challenging it.

The subject of the "DNR" (Do not resuscitate) order may be difficult to discuss, and emotional reactions can be expected. However, the physician should ascertain the family's expectations and desires beforehand rather than learn after the fact that they were dissatisfied with the decision. Usually, the conditions surrounding terminal malignant disease are such that all concerned have ample time and opportunity to come to grips with the issue of the patient's death. When the question of resuscitation arises, the family typically is prepared to deal with it.

The question is often posed whether "DNR" or "No code" orders should be handled orally rather than recorded on the patient's chart. Legal commentators on this subject overwhelmingly favor a written order by the attending physician. Still, some physicians, for one reason or another, are unwilling to commit themselves in writing to this course. Their reticence would seem to be based upon a misplaced fear of the legal consequences. As indicated in the early part of this chapter, the physician usually has no legal duty to render care that is inconsistent with the standards regularly observed by the medical profession. It is quite clear that the profession neither supports nor follows the practice of resuscitating end-stage patients. The "Standards for Cardiopulmonary Resuscitation (CPR) and Emergency Cardiac Care (ECC)," updated in 1980 by the National Academy of Sciences National Research Council, states that CPR is intended to prevent sudden and unexpected death and that it is not indicated "in cases of terminal irreversible illness where death is not unexpected."

In cases in which no legal duty to attempt CPR exists, there is no risk in stating this decision on the patient's permanent record. Properly handled, the notation documents that the resuscitation has been carefully considered in the context of the patient's condition and found to be contraindicated. The patient's record also should indicate that the DNR decision was discussed with the family and that their agreement was obtained.

The Dinnerstein Case

The question of DNR orders was considered in an important 1978 Massachusetts case, *In Re Dinnerstein*,[20] a decision that undermines that state's earlier insistence upon judicial intervention in termination of treatment cases. Two family members, the attending physician, and a hospital representative petitioned a Massachusetts probate court for authorization to enter a DNR order on the chart of a 76-year-old woman who was terminally ill and comatose. A patient advocate was appointed by the court. After hearing both sides, the court ruled that the DNR order was appropriate, stating that the question should be decided by the attending physician in collaboration with the family and in conformity with appropriate medical standards. The ruling made clear that in such cases it is unnecessary to obtain a court's advance authorization for a DNR order. The court would review the physician's decision in these matters only upon a showing that the physician did not act reasonably and in accordance with professional standard principles in deciding not to resuscitate.

Caring for the terminally ill and deciding to withhold or withdraw life support often are difficult. To the extent that the physician fears legal liability from that decision, it is even more troublesome. Fortunately, although the law on this subject is not yet settled, all jurisdictions' legal developments to date have been rational and generally supportive of common medical practice. The law does not expect miraculous cures, nor does it require physicians to proceed as if miracles were possible. Humane, sensitive treatment, rendered with due regard for the patient's right of self-determination, is all that is demanded or expected.

Jurisdictions may provide for certain formalities, such as the execution of a "Natural Death directive" in California. Documentation of the patient's wishes, or those of the next of kin where appropriate, may be advisable to assure legal safety for the health care team. However, note that the ultimate objective of the law in this area is to assure that patients and those close to them are treated with sensitivity and tenderness. To insist upon intrusive formalities for the legal protection of the health care provider when this would further disturb those already in deep distress is unjustified. Humanistic health professionals, assisted by competent legal counsel when appropriate, surely can devise ways to satisfy the formal needs of the situation without placing unnecessary stress upon patients and their loved ones. The end of life should be as free of distress as modern science and old-fashioned compassion can make it.

REFERENCES

1. *Schloendorff v. Society of New York Hospital*, 211 N.Y. 125, 105 N.E. 92,93 (1914).
2. *Salgo v. Leland Stanford, Jr., University Board of Trustees*, 154 Cal. App. 2d 560, 317 P.2d 170 (1957).
3. *Natanson v. Kline*, 187 Kan. 186, 354 P.2d 670 (1960).
4. *Canterbury v. Spence*, 464 F.2d 772 (1972).
5. Id. at 794, n. 138.
6. Id. at 783–4.
7. Id. at 789.
8. *In the Matter of Karen Quinlan, an Alleged Incompetent*, 70 N.J. 10, 355 A.2d 647 (1976).
9. *Roe v. Wade*, 410 U.S. 113 (1973).
10. *In the Matter of Karen Quinlan, an Alleged Incompetent*, 70 N.J. 10 at 41.
11. Raible, "The Right to Refuse Treatment and Natural Death Legislation" 5 *Medicolegal News*, 6,7 (Fall 1977).
12. Papal Allocution to a Congress of Anesthetists (24 November 1957), *Acta Apostolica Sedis* 1027-33 (1957).
13. *Superintendent of Belchertown State School v. Saikewicz*, 370 N.E. 2d 417 (1977).
14. Id. at 430.
15. Id. at 434–5.
16. Sup. Ct., Nassau County, New York, No. 21242-I/79 (Dec. 6, 1979).
17. California Health and Safety Code, § 7185 *et. seq.* (1976).
18. A good review of the California act and provisions of various other states' natural death legislation is the article by Raible, cited above at n. 11.
19. California Health and Safety Code, § 7187(c).
20. 380 N.E. 2d 134 (1978).

Chapter 15

Anthropological Perspectives

Edward L. Schieffelin

Anthropologists do not view the phenomenon of death mainly as a biologic event but as a social one, a human experience reflecting a particular way of life and system of belief. Death may be physically identical in all cultures, but it is by no means the same experience. The shared core of the dying process—the cessation of function of the biologic organism—evokes in the dying individual, his family, and the community a variety of responses which differ according to their cultural orientation. This chapter explores the significance of dying as a cultural event. Further, aspects of death and dying that transcend the medical are considered in order to see what insights a cultural perspective may offer for our own management of dying patients.

DEATH AS TRANSITION AND TRANSFORMATION

Different cultures construct, or constitute, their perceptions of death in different ways. Underlying this diversity of modes of experiencing dying is an archetypal theme that is basic to all human life. This is the theme of transition and transformation. Everywhere, dying represents an ending for the individual and an end of an era for his immediate social group. But this may be viewed variously as a completion or a loss, a climax or a destruction, a disruption or a disappearance, and it nearly always leaves a social vacuum. One who has died does not return. At the same time, his death also appears as a kind of new beginning. For the individual it means a new state of being, whether in an afterlife, in reincarnation, or merely in oblivion. For the community it means a cleansing of the social slate, a movement of succession, a new era, and a new situation for those who cared for the dead person and for his community. It is this *transition*, rather than the "end," from which one cannot return.

Dying is a transition and transformation in and of itself; the passage from one mode of being to another, but as such it is also a fundamental symbol of all transitions/transformations that are experienced in life. In other words, in most cultures, how people understand death also contributes to how they conceptualize, express, and effect important transitions in life. Death is not only a kind of passage itself; it is also the major symbolic mode for expressing and effecting transformations in rites of passage. If we can understand this archetypic transitional significance of death, this may help both dying patients and those who work with them, for the transitional significance is shared on some level by all humankind and has been the basis for much of human art and philosophy.

RITES OF PASSAGE

What is meant by a "rite of passage," and how are we to understand its relationship with death? In 1909 Arnold Van Gennep published a classic work, *Les Rites de Passage*, in which he showed that throughout the world ceremonies marking childbirth, adulthood, newly achieved social status, investment of new leadership, and other important social transitions all had the same internal structure.[1] First, a series of enactments or events occur that serve to separate the individual from his former state or role in life. These are followed by a liminal period, which can be short or long, during which the individual inhabits an anomalous state outside the normal social scheme of his community. It is during this time, when the individual is neither really a member of his society nor yet outside of it, that the transformation in his social state takes place. Often, as Victor Turner has pointed out,[2] this liminal period is marked by reversals of normal social roles, bizarre symbols, and frightening and/or painful ordeals, all of which both destroy the vestiges of the individual's former social role and orientation and prepare him to be reborn a new social person.

Finally, enactments take place that reintegrate the individual into the community, but in a new capacity, role, quality, or position.

Frequently these rites of transition/transformation are formulated overtly or covertly in terms of symbols of death and rebirth: one must die to his old social self, that he may be reborn anew. The paradigmatic case is initiation into adulthood. In tribal societies where this occurs, the initiates (for this discussion, young boys) are separated from their mothers and familiar childhood contexts and taken to a ceremonial place (the bush, the men's house, or the like). By this act the young boy dies, in effect, to his childhood. In keeping with this, mothers frequently wail and mourn their departed sons as they would the dead.

The boys frequently are stripped of their clothing and dressed in special ways that set them apart from and outside of the normal order of society. During this time the initiates learn important cultural information appropriate to maturity. They may be subjected to harsh and traumatic ordeals that prove their courage, force them to submit to the cultural order that is to be their fate in life, and mark them physically (by scarification or circumcision) as new persons. Finally, they are given new vestments, weapons, or ornaments, and are readmitted into society amid celebration as new people who no longer are children to their mothers, but are young men among men. Like one who has died, the initiate cannot return to his former life and state. He is a socially different person, made over, and reborn. Thus, the notions of death and rebirth are the fundamental symbols of transformation that organize the process of social transition. But, as symbols of passage, they bring the notion of passage back to bear upon the problem of the meaning of death itself.

Symbols of transition and transformation and the structure of the passage rite are manifest nearly everywhere in the world in the way people deal with dying and death. At the time of death, the individual, his community, and sometimes the local region of the cosmos are seen to go through a transition, and this transition is marked by the rites accompanying dying and by the funeral. It is in this context that the particular way in which people respond to death and manage the process of passage reveals the meaning that death has for them.

SIGNIFICANCE OF FUNERAL RITES IN DIFFERENT CULTURES

Although funeral rites are all concerned with the transition represented by death, different cultures emphasize different aspects of it because they perceive death in different ways. In some places, funerals emphasize facilitating the journey of the deceased's soul to the afterworld (thus getting it away from the local community where it might cause mischief); elsewhere they concentrate on repairing the social fabric of the community, or on redressing cosmic forces unbalanced by the death event. The diversity of meanings perceived in the situation of dying and death may be illustrated by examining some of the funeral practices of people around the world.

An emphasis on death as completion as well as detachment from (social) life is illustrated by the practices of the Kaliai people of western New Britain, an island in the South Pacific.[3] Here, in a good death the dying person calls together his relatives, debtors, and creditors in the few days before he dies. He settles all of his outstanding debts and relationships so that when the end comes he has few, if any, unfulfilled commitments. Debts are paid; relationships are settled. When he dies, then, ceremony is minimal. In effect, the dying person has completed and disconnected from his life socially before doing so biologically. If he dies prematurely, his relatives settle his affairs, and the funeral is proportionally more elaborate.

Funerals reveal different conceptions of the social self and the relation of individual and community. One set of conceptions, widespread in Papua New Guinea,[4] and among the Bara people of Madagascar[5] concerns ideas about the "biologic" composition of the human body. People in these cultures recognize that an individual is composed of elements deriving partly from the mother and partly from the father. However, it is not our familiar genetic notion of the egg and sperm. Rather, typically, the soft parts of the body, such as the tissues and blood, are felt to come from the mother's side of the family, while the hard parts, or non-bloody parts (the bones and skin), come from the father's side.

In New Guinea this conceptualization is usually based on the correspondence between the red color of the tissues and the mother's menstrual blood on the one hand, and on the white color of bone and the color of semen on the other. The two sides are felt to have contributed equally to the individual, and consequently the father's line must make payments to the mother's people in order to validate their claim to the individual for their group.[4] Another payment is made at the time of death to compensate them for the loss, as well as to effect a quitting of all claims and termination of the relationship that went through him.

Among the Bara of Madagascar, the opposition between the tissues (from the mother) and the bones (from the father) marks a fundamental metaphysical issue in their rational understanding of the world that is deeply implicated in a wide range of activities. The society is patrilineal; the major groups are strongly corporate lineages based on descent from father to son. Social groups are defined in terms of lines of men. Women are seen to enter from the outside by marriage to produce more men, but the enduring feature of the social order, its bones, so to speak, is the male lineage. The permanence of the bones represents not only that part of the body believed to result from the father, but also the enduring quality of the father's lineage. The soft parts of the body, deriving from the mother on the other hand, represent impermanence and decay. They vanish after death as does the relationship with the mother's lineage represented by the dead man himself. At the same time, because bones are durable and because they represent the enduring part of the social organization, they also represent, on a more philosophic level, order as opposed to chaos.

The Bara have a clear notion that order and form are not enough for life, that if everything were strictly ordered, there would be no creative movement at all. Vitality, motion, and activity also are necessary. Thus, at death:

> . . . the dead sterile order of bone is (seen to be) taking dominion over the ebbing vitality of the decomposing flesh. Reality has moved from a state of mediated equilibrium between order and vitality to a state of pure fatal order. This extreme aspect of order. . . can only be opposed by the most extreme aspects of vitality. . . (to restore the balance).[5]

The Bara resolve this problem by staging their funerals as revitalization scenarios. After a period of silence and somber mourning following a death, activities become increasingly festive. Young men and women become sexually provocative towards one another. Laughing, singing, dancing, and wrestling begin, cattle are stampeded, and people get drunk. At the climax, young men shoulder the coffin and race with it in relays to the burial cave, rattling the corpse around in the box. In this way the moribund social area surrounding the death is revitalized and some of that chaotic and unordered vitality is communicated to the corpse itself as it is jostled in the coffin and the spirit makes its way home to be with the ancestors.

The relationship between the individual, the community, and death has a different quality among the Kaluli people of Papua New Guinea.[6] Here the social emphasis in the process of dying is

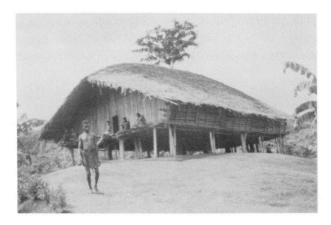

Fig. 15–1. Kaluli longhouse of Clan Wabisi at Tusuku.

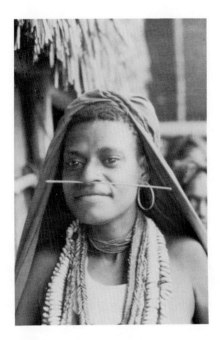

Fig. 15–2. Kaluli woman.

one of fear (of others in the manner of dying), and of grief and rage at the loss. This is frequently followed by vengeance.

The Kaluli people live in isolated longhouses in a dense tropical forest north of Mount Bosavi on the Papuan Plateau (Figs. 15–1 and 15–2.)

Each community consists of about 60 people, or roughly 15

families. Traditionally these people were subject to raids from their neighbors, and therefore they have built their longhouses high on posts as fortresses against this eventuality. Peaceful relations are maintained by intermarriage between communities and by ceremonial gifts of food exchanged between in-laws, friends, and relatives.

The Kaluli believe in a reasonably pleasant afterlife in a spirit world following death. However, this plays relatively little part in their management of dying or of death. The Kaluli believe that all deaths without exception, and including death by accident and deaths in fights, are caused by witches. A witch is a person with an evil substance or creature in his heart. While the witch sleeps, this creature creeps out invisibly, takes the form of his host while remaining invisible, and wanders about in a Dracula-like fashion seeking prey.

His victim awakes the next day with a high fever and the physical disability of severe illness. If a spirit medium is called in, he frequently finds that the witch has cut off his victim's legs (or rather their invisible counterpart), which explains why the patient is unable to get up and walk. Alternatively, the witch may have put a stone in his throat whence he cannot swallow. If not stopped, the witch later returns to carry off additional body parts while the victim weakens and eventually, when his heart is removed (invisibly), he dies. Here the experience of dying is rather horrific, infused with paranoid fear that someone else is "getting you." In the altered state of consciousness of approaching death, when patients are already partly in the invisible world, they commonly can "see" the witch approaching, even though no else can.

Picture the impact of this experience on the dying scene: Typically one finds the dying individual lying with his head on the lap of one of his relatives with others gathered around apprehensively attending to him and vainly hoping that their presence will keep witches away. As the patient nears death, relatives may urge him to speak the name of his invisible attacker, and occasionally this becomes a dramatic, terrifying scene if the dying person thinks he sees the witch approaching. He starts up, wide-eyed with fear, staring at an unseen presence: "Look there! He's coming in the door!" Those gathered round him look about and see no one. However, they all know well what is happening. The senior man or closest relative will urge "Who is it? Tell us who it is!" The dying person sinks back in horror and gasps: "He is taking my heart!" "Who is it? Who is it?" his relatives repeat, and the patient finally

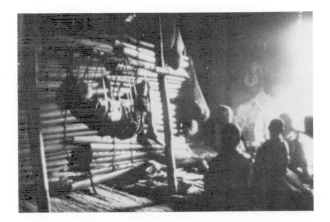

Fig. 15–3. Women mourners attending the corpse in the longhouse.

manages to speak a name. Soon thereafter he collapses and dies while his relatives break into loud wails of grief.

Not all Kaluli deaths are this dramatic, although the sick become increasingly apprehensive and jumpy as they worsen. Nevertheless, the occasional dramatic death like this serves as a paradigm for the Kaluli conception of what dying is about. It is an eerie and awful way to die.

The matter, of course, does not end here. While the dead makes his way to the spirit world (a journey itself conceived in terms of passage and rebirth), his friends and relatives grieve, smolder with anger, and thirst for revenge against the witch who did him in. The corpse is suspended from a log in cane loops and hung inside the longhouse. Two small fires keep down the stench of decomposition as relatives from surrounding longhouses come to mourn, members of a different community arriving each day in succession (Figs. 15–3 and 15–4).

This is more than the simple funeral viewing that we have in our own society. It has more sinister implications. The witch responsible for the death often does not know of his responsibility because his witch aspect usually operates while he is asleep. If he shows up unwittingly with the other mourners during the funeral period, the body is said to suddenly move or discharge fluids identifying his presence in the crowd and enabling steps toward revenge to begin.

After three or four days when all of the visitors have paid their respects or the stench has become too unpleasant, the body is removed from the house and placed in a raised exposed coffin

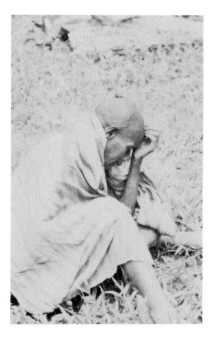

Fig. 15–4.   A mother mourns her daughter.

some distance from the dwelling (Fig. 15–5). If the individual was important or especially beloved, the bones later may be recovered and hung in a net bag in a dry place under the eaves of the longhouse as a sentimental gesture. Meanwhile, the desire for revenge remains. Shortly after the funeral, divinations are performed to confirm the identity of the witch responsible. Once confirmation is established and if people still feel strongly enough about the death, a raiding party is organized. The longhouse of the witch is surrounded just before dawn. The door is opened by treachery, and the raiders rush in, grab the witch, and club him to death. At this point the relatives and friends of the murdered witch are aroused. The raiders must quickly drag the body outside and perform an autopsy, while holding off the dead man's relatives, to prove by certain internal signs that he really was a witch. If proof is sufficient the inhabitants of the longhouse accept his guilt and abide by the justice of revenge. Nevertheless, they themselves have sustained a loss and demand payment of compensation. When this is made, peace is restored.

     Not every Kaluli death is avenged. The number of raids feasible within a particular span of time is self-limiting due to the

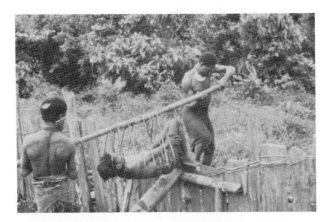

Fig. 15–5.   Removing the corpse to the exposed coffin.

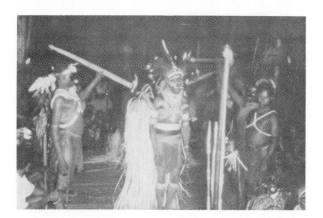

Fig. 15–6.   Gisalo dancer.

tensions and divisions aroused by murders within and between communities. Consequently, revenge killings happen only about 10% of the time. Nevertheless, anger and revenge are implications that underlie every death, and contemplations on the tragedy of loss through death, the experience of grief, anger, and violence, and the payment of compensation constitute the major themes of the highest forms of Kaluli poetic and dramatic art.[5]

Kaluli do not memorialize their dead through monuments or carvings. Rather, they remember them in their songs and dances. In their major ceremony, called Gisalo, beautifully decorated dancers sing songs that subtly allude to the dead (Fig. 15–6).[6]

Members of the audience become deeply moved and burst into

tears. Then, their sadness turning to rage, they retaliate for their grief by scorching the dancer on the shoulder blades with torches. The dancer continues as if he feels no pain, but after the ceremony, he pays small items of compensation to those in the audience whom he caused to weep. Thus he not only reevokes the memory of the dead, but also enables the people to express their grief and anger and to be compensated for their sense of loss. The drama and tragedy of death thus is rearoused and re-resolved.

These ceremonies, despite their emotional and even violent content, are expressions of intimacy among people who are closely allied. They are never given at funerals, but occur rather at festive occasions of prestation (customary gift-giving between in-laws or kinsmen) and marriage between friendly groups, and are part of the acknowledgment of intimacy and trust between them. At the same time, the ceremonies reflect the shadow of grief, loneliness, fear, and violence that death casts over the lives of all.

AMERICAN FUNERAL PRACTICES

The way that death is dealt with in other societies has been described in order to show how it varies across cultures in meaning, in how it is experienced, and in its outcome. The purpose also has been to show the ways in which death involves the passage scenario for the dead himself and for the community as a whole, although different aspects of the passage are emphasized in different places. For the Kaluli, the retaliation scenario—whether carried out directly in the killing of a witch or vicariously in ceremonial performance—revitalizes and redresses those who have suffered the loss, and allows them to resolve their anger and vengefulness.

What light does this throw on our own American ways of death? What insight does it give that can be employed to help the dying? What can we understand about the significance of death to Americans as reflected in our own death rituals? Huntington and Metcalf point out:

> Given the many varieties of death rites throughout the world and the cultural heterogeneity of American society, the expectation is that funeral practices will vary widely from one region, or social class, or ethnic group, to another. The odd fact is that they do not. The overall form of funerals is remarkably uniform from coast to coast.[5]

Most Americans are given a funeral that involves speedy removal of the body from the place of death to the funeral parlor, where it is embalmed, powdered, and painted with cosmetics to make it look alive. It is then laid in a comfortable casket to be viewed by relatives. This is followed by its removal to the cemetery for final interment. The entire process is rather rapid compared to the five-day Kaluli funeral or to funeral celebrations elsewhere that continue for weeks or even months.

Sometimes criticized for ostentation, the American-style funeral service and the cortege of cars led by a hearse actually are quite subdued compared to the singing, dancing, wrestling, and sexual license among the Bara. American funerals certainly are less expensive and ostentatious than those in which huge catafalques are carried in procession by up to 30 men, as seen in the funerals in Bali, or those in which large-scale public death payments are accompanied by the slaughter of pigs, as is done in the Melanesian Islands.[7]

Doubtless the fact that funeral directing is a profit-making business is partially responsible for the standardization of American funerals, as Mitford argues.[8] However, it is equally clear that funeral parlors could not successfully remain in business if the way they handled death did not reflect on some level the fundamental needs and beliefs of contemporary American culture. Although diversity of ethnic background and religious belief is reflected in the variety of religious services and in other funeral details, the basic form remains the same. In particular, the treatment of the body says a great deal about the way Americans feel about death, regardless of their background. The body is embalmed to preserve it, but not necessarily permanently. What is important is its cosmetic appearance. The purpose of American-style cosmetic embalming is to enable others to view the dead person looking as though he were healthy and asleep, with a serene, contented countenance.

Critics of this form of funeral practice such as Becker[9] and Bowman[10] claim that it documents American's underlying fear of death and represents an attempt to deny death by making the corpse appear alive. Although the tendency to shy away from confrontation with mortality is an undeniable feature of American society[5], the beautified corpse also may be expressing a positive statement about the American attitude toward death. This is the desire to see in death not merely an end, but a sense of completion—a sense that the person has been freed from the cares of life or the pain and disfigurement of illness and that he is serene now in death, resting peacefully as in the transformation from wakefulness to sleep.

The final image, then, projected by the carefully prepared body itself, is of the person in the *spiritual* state that he and his loved ones would want him to inhabit. His relatives know that he is not alive, but they do want him to be free of the signs of corruption, disease, pain, or unhappiness, especially if these signs have marked his last days. They want to think of him as beyond all that now and in repose, having lived a complete life.

Without any explicit suggestion of an afterlife, the American corpse projects the implication that the individual has passed into some other—probably better—state of being. This implication is consistent with most religious faiths, and with the agnosticism of contemporary pluralistic American society.

The common theme and structure of transition/transformation run through the varied responses to death that have been discussed. The major difference between death and other transitions is that death represents for the individual not a transition from one stage of life to another, but a transition out of life altogether. Nevertheless, the structure of passage is based upon the notion of dying and death, followed by transformation and rebirth, as archetypal symbols of transformation in life. This may help us to provide meaningful guidance for those going through the experience of dying.

FACTORS INFLUENCING QUALITY OF DEATH IN AMERICA

Several demographic and epidemiologic characteristics of dying in the United States contribute to its special qualities, and hence to the particular problems that dying patients and their caregivers face here. People in most of the non-Western cultures discussed do not have access to Western-type medical facilities, and the life span among them rarely exceeds 50 or 55 years. Moreover, most people die of infectious disorders with fairly rapid courses. Consequently, there are few dependent or feeble elderly people in these societies, and long-lingering terminal illnesses are rare.

In America, the reverse is true. Medical therapy, skillful nursing, and high technology life-support systems have resulted in a situation in which people can expect to die at a comparatively advanced age. Moreover, those who die in hospitals frequently do so after comparatively lengthy illnesses. The dying individual under these circumstances faces a period of increasing debility and dependence in a society that values independence and vigor, with no hope at the end but death. Lying in a hospital and inhabiting the transitional state of dying, the individual is in a situation analogous to that of the initiate, who, removed from the village and stripped of his clothing and individuality, looks anxiously toward the relatively unknown but frequently fearsome and painful ordeals he knows he must face; ordeals that will change him for the rest of his life. But in a large, impersonal hospital where the dying patient all too frequently may be left alone, the individual finds himself abandoned. He is like the initiate without an initiator to guide, instruct, or support his passage, or to help him understand the meaning of his ordeal.

Death, like initiation, is implicitly a social rather than an individual phenomenon for human beings. Death always occurs in the context of others. Whether the patient is surrounded or abandoned by loved ones, whether he is mourned or ignored, his death is always understood as a human death in relation to absent and present others. It cannot be morally ignored. Doctors and nurses who attend the dying preside over an area that, unlike the curing of illness, is not, strictly speaking, a medical function; it is a priestly, or even a shamanic function. Those who preside over the transition between life and death fulfill a role that, like initiation, implicitly is infused with a certain sacred quality. It is not surprising that this role should sit uneasily on the shoulders of scientific medicine. This is partly because medical people do not see the sacred as their domain. But, in addition, practitioners of Western medicine see their role in therapy as negotiating the transition from illness to health, in other words, producing cure. From this perspective, death represents failure, and failure is especially disturbing if it is preceded by heroic efforts.

For this and other reasons, medical professionals, like other Americans, often shy away from the inevitability of mortality as represented in the person of the terminally ill patient. Those caring for the dying must try to understand the degree to which their roles are more than medical. Inevitably, medical professionals are guides in a process of passage who are called upon not only to comfort the dying, but also to help them find their way toward meaning.

In our desacralized and skeptical society it is difficult to know how caregivers can deal with roles that seem to encompass a sacred domain. We have for the most part lost any clear sense of an afterlife to which death is the gateway and passage. In such a situation, an anthropologist tends to look to the meanings expressed in art and ritual to see in what direction the deepest collective insights of a culture point. If we look therefore at our own funerals, and in particular at the symbolism of the body which expresses the significance of the death upon the individual himself, we see what Americans in some sense wish for or feel is appropriate at the end of the trajectory of life.

Whatever may be inferred about an afterlife, a sense of completedness, serenity, and repose is represented bodily as the final hoped-for spiritual condition. The task of mediating and guiding the final transition, therefore, is not simply that of making a patient comfortable. The task includes guiding him and helping him attain, as best one can, that final internal serenity and sense of completion represented by our ritual preparation of the body.

This points to a task well beyond palliative care to ameliorate physical suffering. It implies active spiritual or psychologic care to help dying people make the passage; to help them find their own way through fear, doubt, pain, and sense of dependency to a final acceptance and peace of mind. This is a task that caregivers increasingly recognize as relevant and necessary, not only for the sake of the dying, but for their own inner humanity and that of all of us as well.

REFERENCES

1. Van Gennep, A.: Les Rites de Passage. Paris, Emile Nourry, 1909.
2. Turner, V.: The Ritual Process. New York, Aldine, 1969.
3. Counts, D.R.: The good death in Kaliai: preparation for death in western New Britain. *In* Death & Dying: Views from Many Cultures. Pespectives on Death and Dying. Vol. I. Edited by Richard A. Kalish. Farmingdale, N.Y., Baywood Publishing Co., 39–44, 1980.
4. Wagner, R.: The Curse of Souw. Chicago, University of Chicago Press, 1967.
5. Huntington, R., and Metcalf, P.: Celebrations of Death: The Anthropology of Mortuary Ritual. New York, Cambridge University Press, 1979.
6. Schieffelin, E.L.: The Sorrow of the Lonely and the Burning of the Dancers. New York, St. Martin's Press, 1976.
7. Malinowski, B.: Argonauts of the Western Pacific. New York, E.P. Dutton & Co., 1922.
8. Mitford, J.: The American Way of Death. New York, Simon & Schuster, 1963.
9. Becker, E.: The Denial of Death. New York, Free Press, 1973.
10. Bowman, L.: The American Funeral: A Study of Guilt, Extravagance and Sublimity. New York, Paperback Library, 1964.

Chapter **16**

Spiritual and Religious Aspects

The Reverend John B. Pumphrey

TERMINAL ILLNESS AND SPIRITUAL NEEDS

Terminal illness can be the occasion for anxious reflection that results in troubled believing, or in what is commonly called a crisis of faith. When the balance of emotional and physical well-being is tipped in favor of disorder and disunity, spiritual well-being is equally challenged. Questions of meaning and purpose arise, often accompanied by feelings of guilt about the past and insecurity about the future. Loss, or its anticipation, is paradigmatic for the existential experience of the "why me?" questioning of God or gods, of fate, or of the universe itself.

Spirituality is rooted in a matrix of meaning and purpose arising from what is termed by some a worldview, by others a philosophy, and by still others, a specific theology. Having "faith" and "believing" are integral processes in one's spiritual economy just as proscriptions and prescriptions are with regard to behavior. Recognizing the spiritual needs of terminal patients, therefore, first entails taking the long or larger view of what is involved for the whole person. It also necessitates becoming attuned to specific signals and symptoms, both positive and negative. We can, for example, be alert to signals that indicate that patients are experiencing a loss of meaning or are undergoing a life review which engenders the need for a sense of forgiveness. These are not simply emotional crises—they can also evidence spiritual and religious need.[1]

Spiritual needs of patients are as diverse as patients themselves. Care must be taken to understand this concept broadly, as the preceding comments imply. For example, not every patient's system of belief involves a relationship with a personal deity. However, the word "spiritual" indicates a quality of dynamic relationship, whether this be, for example, a relationship with a cause, with a group, or with realities identified as beyond or above the natural. Spiritual needs can and do arise when this relationship is threatened or when the relationship itself is shattered.

Spiritual needs may become manifest in overt behaviors such as talking about God, reading religious literature, questioning the purpose of suffering, or requesting a chaplain to visit. Certain occasions during illness tend to give rise to questioning or conflict: the time of diagnosis; initial hospitalization; pretreatment decision-making; anticipated loss of body parts; and impending death. Any conflict that erupts in the course of illness, such as financial or family difficulties, may be colored by ethical and moral interpretations based upon a person's theology. Even patients who seem overtly hostile to religion may experience anxiety regarding their spiritual needs.

Based upon earlier work of Allport,[2,4] studies have differentiated between extrinsically and intrinsically supported belief. Extrinsically supported belief, or religious orientation, finds its source in custom or peer pressure. It is far less likely to prove helpful in times of crisis, particularly during the crisis of terminal illness, than an orientation more central to the basic core of one's personality and background. Yet even an internalized, integrated religious orientation, or intrinsically supported belief, does not exempt one from difficulty, trauma, crisis, and accompanying doubts. The professed believer is subject to the same assaults that others may experience and perhaps to a greater need to resolve doubts when they occur.

Response to crisis in general, and to terminal illness in particular, is to some extent guided or circumscribed by cultural expectations. Changes have occurred in our society regarding our ability to conceive of a providential god, for example. We no longer have the significant and ongoing sense of relationship to transcendental realities that prevailed in the nineteenth century.[5] There has been a dramatic transition away from nineteenth century theology and toward a heroic humanism; toward a focus on individualism that instructs us to accept dying, to go out smiling, and to fulfill our jobs and responsibilities up to the very end. These are our contemporary values. Sometimes the discrepancy between cultural norms and expectations on the one hand, and one's personal needs or predispositions on the other, exacerbates the spiritual crisis and impedes the patient's ability to adjust. Recognizing terminal patients' spiritual needs and conflicts is essential to good care. In attending to these needs we acknowledge implicitly their impact on the patient's response to proposed or ongoing treatment regimens, as well as their impact on the doctor-patient relationship.

HOW THE CLINICIAN CAN HELP

Patients require recognition of their spiritual concerns. Even more, they require understanding responses from those who provide their medical care. Health professionals neither need to be experts in religion nor need to be particularly anxious when faced with patients' spiritual needs and religious practices. Sensitivity to individual differences, a willingness for open inquiry, and a readiness for frank discussion will guide the practitioner in this as in any other area of care.

It is often difficult for health professionals to discuss spiritual concerns. Our own biases, anxieties, self-projections, or personal systems of belief may inhibit the possibility of dialogue, although the patient may very much desire dialogue on this subject. Even socially intimate relationships often exclude a meaningful exchange of views aimed at mutual understanding of religious belief and practice. Friends share their views on sex and their deepest fears about physical illness and death itself. Emotional vulnerability and availability are declared essential elements of satisfactory interpersonal relationships. "God talk," however, is often considered too private a subject for discussion. Religion may be the last taboo, replacing the subjects of death and sex in this respect.

Inquiry following observed behavior, then, is an important acknowledgment that a patient's concerns, including spiritual concerns, are heard and respected. Such an inquiry also demonstrates a willingness to try to understand even a system of belief or practice different from one's own. Care must be taken that the patient does not perceive inquiry and subsequent dialogue about spiritual and religious matters as one of the "last things" that must be attended to. The matter of timing, of when to discuss significant areas of concern, requires careful judgment and individual consideration.

Concluding that a patient's spiritual concerns and religious practices are, or should be, off limits can also arise from a nagging sense of incompetence and a desire to flee from matters of theology and faith. The physician or other health professional is not expected to have answers where none exist. Dialogue does require a measure of self-disclosure and honesty, and a willingness to express opinion or belief when appropriate. The focus of discussion, however, should remain the patient's concerns. Listening is more helpful than trying to resolve issues or reassure too quickly.

Some patients try to present the impression that everything is fine and that their "house" is in order. Patients, of course, live and die by the cultural norms and expectations noted earlier. Although patients certainly are entitled to their privacy, even the most stoic among them may desire and appreciate the opportunity to discuss their emotional and spiritual responses to illness and impending death. Clinicians are accustomed to sensitive physical examination and to exploration of mental and emotional states. They can apply this same sensitivity with equally fruitful results to inquiry about and sharing of spiritual concerns.

A particular problem for many clinicians is how to respond to religious phenomena that patients say they experience. There is no easy answer here, and to some extent the matter turns upon the level of conflict or pain induced, or upon the extent to which interpersonal relationships are disrupted. However, while you or I may not be able to see angels or perceive our sickness as a gift from God, some patients do, and the result for them may be comfort and solace as opposed to conflict and pain. Healing, even in the face of terminal illness, takes many forms.

PRAYER AND RELIGIOUS RITUAL

Attending to the spiritual dimension of care along with those of the body and mind is less difficult and problematic than it often appears. An appreciation of the role of prayer and religious ritual also helps the health professional's assessment of and intervention in the patient's care. Prayer is a very personal form of communication to many. It also may be communal and formalized through worship. When the person prays, alone or in community, a relationship to God is acknowledged and intended. The use of words or verbalizing is normative but not required for prayer. Both Western and Eastern traditions encompass the practice of contemplation and meditation that does not require the use of words. Whatever the modality, prayer is a conscious and deliberate action on the part of believers to open themselves to the presence and power of God in their lives.[6]

Patients' prayers may express fear and anger; lament; joy and thanksgiving; and petition and intercession, particularly that healing may occur. One must realize that religious persons do not always perceive physical healing as the ultimate manifestation of God's love or regard for them. Many patients, including terminal patients, can and do experience profound changes in their attitudes and responses to suffering through prayer. Patients frequently report a sense of peace attained through prayer after a period of emotional turmoil and physical pain.

Rituals are actions that tend to rule in and/or rule out important elements of behavior, attitude, or belief within the individual and community of believers. Religious rituals performed in times of crisis or transition fulfill the important function of maintenance and reparation in relationship to divine realities. Patients may interpret their illness in a variety of ways, viewing it, for example, as a punishment, as a teaching experience, as a means of purification, or as a sacrifice on behalf of another. Therefore, rituals associated with reconciliation and forgiveness become vitally important.[6] Rituals involving a sense of becoming incorporated, or "at-one" with God or with the divine, may become a necessary next step. Participation in the ritual of Holy Communion contains this aspect for many. Ritual actions employ profound symbols for the believer; the ritual of Holy Communion in its use of bread is a significant example. Bread is a powerful symbol of life, and for many believers it is a reminder of God's will for them even beyond physical death.

Many rituals are specifically intended for healing, such as anointing with oil and the laying on of hands. Without arguing the efficacy of these actions for physical healing, we must realize that they do serve the important purpose for the believer of placing the whole of one's self, body, mind, and spirit, in the care of God.

Religious rituals and prayer thus provide patients with a significant means of care and, frequently, of hope. By their very nature, they invite patients into relationships beyond themselves even while permitting solitary expression. Clinicians will recognize in these manifestations of a person's spirituality a positive contribution to their patient's adaptation to terminal illness in particular. Yet sensitive clinicians will not view prayer and ritual too narrowly as "resources," analogous to instruments or medications. Rather they will regard patients' participation in ritual as a personal statement of who they are as persons.

COLLABORATION WITH CLERGY

In addition to the clinician's personal initiative and sensitive response, the clergy's assistance may prove invaluable to intervention and care. Many patients have a relationship with a member of the clergy. Their minister, priest, or rabbi already may be involved in their care, or may be readily responsive to the needs of family members. Inquiry here will help assess the importance and extent of the ongoing pastoral care relationship, and it can determine the need or desire for renewed or additional contact with clergy. If no relationship with a member of the clergy exists, referral to a hospital chaplain may be in order. Many institutions, even those lacking a formal department of pastoral care, have contacts with community clergy who are willing volunteers for just such occasions.

Some hospitals have their own chaplains who can assist directly in care, make needed referrals, or work in close association with the patient's own pastor. Many if not most full-time hospital chaplains today are well trained and qualified to serve in health care settings. They are graduates of seminaries or schools of religion, and also have received the clinical training necessary for their function as spiritual counselors during the time of illness. Many chaplains have additional training that certifies them professionally in secular disciplines of counseling. The professional chaplain or pastoral counselor may be certified to function specifically in this role by such organizations as the College of Chaplains, a division of the American Protestant Hospital Association; the Association for Clinical Pastoral Education; or the American Association of Pastoral Counselors.

Chaplains or clergy, thus trained and certified, are familiar with the clinical setting. They are particularly sensitive to and capable of dealing with grief, and dying surely is a grief experience. Hospital chaplains know firsthand the patient's problems and response to illness, and they are aware of the dynamics and demands upon the health care team. Clergy who are also trained counselors can see a person's religious belief in the context of other relevant concerns. They are therefore potential allies in the care of the patient's emotional, spiritual, and religious needs. The chaplain, for example, may be the most appropriate person to call upon for help in assessing a religious phenomenon experienced by a patient or in determining the need for psychiatric evaluation. The chaplain, by training and experience, can be an important resource for both patients and staff.

Principles of good referral apply to the clergy as to other consultants. Preferably, discussion should take place with the patient prior to the referral and should cover the reasons for requesting the chaplain's visit. It might be explained that you or others feel inadequately trained to deal with religious or spiritual concerns, but that a chaplain is available. Sufficient advance information should be provided to the chaplain to assist pastoral assessment and care. Any changes in behavior or attitude should be noted, as should evidence of interpersonal conflict that may impinge upon care and the course of treatment. Such information helps the chaplain, even if no particular problem has been identified.

The clinician should expect to receive, from the chaplain in particular, a written or verbal report describing at least the initial encounter with the patient, within the bounds of confidentiality of the chaplain-patient relationship. The clinician may also contact the patient's own clergy to exchange information and to develop mutually supportive efforts in caregiving. This, of course, should be done with the patient's awareness and permission.

RELIGION AND DYING

The intrinsic or extrinsic character of a person's spirituality and religious practice influences the quality and character of his dying. Where religion has contributed to the ability to trust; where meaning and purpose have been enhanced, if not established, in and through believing; where life's ambiguities are dealt with realistically; and where a sense of providential, transcendental care has been maintained, adjustment to dying often is easier. However, peace and tranquility are not the guaranteed results of religious belief; nor should peace and tranquility, explicitly or implicitly, be expected of those who have openly declared their faith. Human frailty is acknowledged by the major faiths of the world, a point that often is forgotten.

Some people react to the prospect of their dying with relative ease, with a spirit of quiet resignation and a sense of summing up or even consummating their lives. Faith and believing may or may not have a role in this response. Others react with a kind of impatience. It is as though, at a point in their pilgrimage toward death, they are more determined than ever to cross over to the other side where they shall see their God face to face. Others are plagued with fear, anxiety, and despair throughout their experience. Such people are not necessarily nonreligious; in fact, they may be quite religious. For them, fuel may be added to their fears by an expectation of punishment for sin. When patients believe that their pain, suffering, and dying are punishments, they have their own reasons for justifying this belief, and sometimes the issue of neurotic as opposed to real guilt is best left moot.

Belief in an afterlife can be a factor in patients' response to dying. Such beliefs take many forms, reflecting the fact that primitive and modern religions throughout the world share notions or expectations of some "life" beyond death. The scriptural heritage underlying the Judeo-Christian tradition, for example, contains little that specifically describes life after death. What is communicated is the promise of God for a continued relationship. Perhaps the nature and content of belief in life after death are of less immediacy than is its clinical impact. One need not feel compelled to intervene with regard to a person's conception of afterlife unless it causes pain or conflict.

The following case history illustrates many of the points introduced in this chapter.

Mr. T. was a 45-year-old married man with two children. He was a successful businessman, having turned a small business into a million-dollar operation. He was intelligent, articulate, and regarded by his friends and colleagues as a man of wit and sensitivity. Mr. T responded to his diagnosis of metastatic cancer of the prostate by challenging the disease almost on a personal basis. He consumed facts concerning his disease and its treatment and demanded that his physician and caregivers tell him everything. He engaged caregivers in profoundly personal ways with his openness to his own and others' feelings.

During one hospitalization some six to eight months after treatment began, Mr. T. became increasingly withdrawn and openly hostile. This marked change in his behavior was assumed to be a normal response to a discouraging course of treatment. He was observed for possible psychiatric intervention. When his behavior persisted, a psychiatrist was called for consultation. Psychiatric findings showed evidence of reactive depression, and a trial of anti-depressant medication was recommended. This note appeared on the written consult:

Patient reports conflicted feelings concerning his religious belief and "faith."

Although Mr. T.'s mood subsequently improved, his personal relationships continued to be strained. At the oncology section team meeting, Mr. T.'s progress and treatment were discussed. The head nurse expressed concern about the psychiatrist's notation of religious conflict. Mr. T. had not expressed concerns in this area previously. Staff was divided over whether and how to intervene. Mr. T.'s physician ended the debate by stating that he would have his own pastor call on Mr. T.

Mr. T. received the pastor's visit cordially but guardedly. Later he spoke with his physician, thanking him for his interest, but requesting that the pastor not visit again.

Two days later, however, Mr. T. did request that a visit be made by the rabbi assigned to the hospital's chaplaincy. The rabbi learned that Mr. T.'s parents had changed their name to hide their Jewish identity when the family moved to another state. Mr. T., then age 11, was not permitted to associate with Jews thereafter. He had "adjusted" to life passing as a nominal Christian without affiliation.

At the time of his diagnosis and illness, Mr. T.'s wife was active in a local parish and began to insist that he attend church and healing services. He had never revealed his background to his wife, and found himself in continual turmoil because of his "lived lie" and his inability to resolve conflicts within himself concerning his own faith orientation.

Extensive contacts with the rabbi enabled Mr. T. to share his religious history with his wife, to express his fears of rejection by her, and gradually to reclaim his identity as a Jew. He wife was helped by both the rabbi and by her own pastor to accept her husband's needs.

At his death both the rabbi and the wife's pastor participated in the funeral service.

This case is not as unusual as it may at first appear. Many critical moments in the lives of patients are associated with some religious event in their upbringing related to specific parental practice. Differences in religious orientation in a marriage can lead to conflict or disappointed expectation. In addition, of course, the experience of illness itself is interpreted and integrated by many through a religious or spiritual perspective. The events described in the example of Mr. T. are unsurprising. A good outcome cannot always be expected, however, and there was no assurance that this would be so for Mr. T. That the outcome in his case was positive was not guaranteed by any disciplined attention to his spiritual concerns, which is the typical approach to this area of care.

The example of Mr. T. illustrates some common features of problem-solving in the clinical arena: observation, evaluation and interpretation, documentation, and intervention. Documentation played a crucial role here. The psychiatrist's notation of the patient's religious concerns made it possible for an alert head nurse to act on the perceived problem. Pastoral involvement of both hospital- and community-based clergy resulted in resolution of major conflict for this patient and prevented painful disruption of intimate relationships at the close of his life. Not only Mr. T. but his wife as well was assisted, and she too was enabled to feel a deep sense of personal satisfaction and peace.

Some real and potential difficulties are also illustrated, such as the danger of making inappropriate assumptions. Mr. T.'s withdrawal was thought to be "normal" in the absence of gross psychiatric pathology and in the face of imminent death. Fortunately, the psychiatrist uncovered the fact that a religious conflict existed. Had this problem been ignored on the assumption that the matter was too private for intervention, the outcome probably would have been less satisfactory.

The physician's use of his own pastor was fraught with difficulties. The patient may have felt pressured to respond to his physician's pastor. In addition, the physician did not first discuss with Mr. T. the suitability of this pastor's visit. The physician is advised to use so close a personal relationship with great care. Professionals are available for consultation and referral, and this route keeps personal bias to a minimum.

This example illustrates both process and system in the approach to patients' spiritual and religious concerns and suggests the important personal dynamics that permeate this experience. Physicians and other health professionals on more than one occasion will be called upon to share themselves, quite often in personal ways.

In summary, it is helpful for the clinician to explore those personal factors that operate to inhibit understanding of and response to spiritual and religious aspects of care. The use of one's powers of observation and judgment are as critical here as in other areas of care. By recognizing the need for frank dialogue and by demonstrating a willingness to understand, the clinician communicates respect for this important dimension of the whole person. The use of clergy, trained hospital chaplains, or clinical ministers is a valuable interdisciplinary approach to care of the dying. Above all else, however, the physician or other health professional should recognize the rich personal rewards possible in such caring. Patients' unique responses to illness and dying demonstrate a characteristic of courage that lies at the heart of mankind and that offers the rest of us hope for the future.

REFERENCES

1. Pumphrey, J.B.: Recognizing your patient's spiritual needs. Nurs., 77:64–68, December, 1977.
2. Allport, B.: The Nature of Prejudice. New York, Doubleday, 1958.
3. Feagin, J.R.: Prejudice and religious types: a focused study of southern fundamentalists. J. Sci. Stud. Religion, 4:3–13, 1964.
4. Magni, K.G.: The fear of death. *In* Death and Presence. Edited by A. Godin. Brussels, Lumen Vitae Press, 1972.
5. Gerkin, C.V.: Crisis Experience in Modern Life. Nashville, Abingdon Press, 1979.
6. Sevensky, R.L.: Religion and illness: an outline of their relationship. South. Med. J., 74:745–750, 1981.

Chapter 17

Symptom Control Manual

Michael H. Levy

Central to the success of palliative care is skilled control of physical symptoms. Consistent with Maslow's hierarchy of needs, physical distress must be alleviated before psychosocial and spiritual pains can be approached and managed successfully. The goal of care for the terminally ill is to optimize the quality of remaining life.

The symptom control techniques presented in this manual may be used for patients for whom disease-oriented therapy is still taking place as well as for those for whom continuation of such therapy is no longer useful or appropriate. Once the underlying disease process becomes irreversible or uncontrollable, certain therapeutic limits and contraindications become less relevant. Narcotic masking of diagnostically important pain or steroid-induced immunosuppression, for example, are of minimal concern in patients with unresponsive, progressive, terminal disease.

Palliative care is active care. It is a form of intensive care, requiring constant reassessment of therapeutic efficacy and toxicity. Until the last few hours of life, most patients require more rather than less therapeutic intervention. When the underlying disease process cannot be controlled, the most minor symptom becomes magnified and demands rapid and skilled control.

PAIN   Pain, the most common physical symptom of terminally ill patients, afflicts 70 to 75% of such patients. Pain control is the most studied and best developed palliative care modality. Nevertheless, for many dying patients in this country, pain relief is far from optimal,

suffering from both inadequate professional knowledge and improper application of current knowledge.

Most terminally ill patients have chronic rather Chronic
than acute pain. Acute pain usually is reversible, linear Pain
(it begins and ends), and meaningful (it is protective,
a warning to seek aid, or a sign of healing). Chronic
pain, conversely, usually is irreversible, intractable,
cyclic, progressive, meaningless, hopeless, and all-con-
suming. Its anticipated perpetuation leads to fear,
anxiety, depression, and a feeling of helplessness that
further worsens the pain perceived and can totally
occupy its victim.

The palliative care plan must encompass patients' Total
psychologic, social, spiritual, and financial "pains" along Pain
with their physical pain. Problems in each of these
areas affect the pain threshold and often require specific, concomitant therapy to achieve adequate control
of physical pain.

Most pains have a constellation of characteristics Pain
that are peculiar to their underlying pathophysiology Evaluation
and thus are helpful in delineating therapy: site,
intensity, quality, variation, and response to prior
therapy.

Pain can be in one site or in several; it can be Site
stationary or radiating. Body diagrams often are useful in delineating the site (simple outlines, dermatome
maps, or organ diagrams).

Reliable, reproducible pain measurement is Intensity
needed to gauge therapeutic efficacy. The three most
commonly used scales follow:

Five-point scales   pain
   0   no pain   measurement
   1   mild   scales
   2   moderate/discomforting
   3   severe/distressing
   4   very severe/horrible
   5   overwhelming/excruciating

Visual analogue scale

No pain
at all _____ / _____ imaginable

Worst pain

Patient's Mark

McGill-Melzack Pain Questionnaire (see Figure 17–1)

Patient's Name_____Date_____Time_____am/pm
Analgesic(s) _____Dosage_____Time Given_____am/pm
_____.Dosage_____Time Given_____am/pm

Analgesic Time Difference (hours): +4 +1 +2 +3
PRI: S_____ A_____ E_____ M(S)_____ M(AE)_____ M(T)_____ PRI(T)_____
    (1-10)   (11-15) (16)   (17-19)   (20)   (17-20) (1-20)

1 FLICKERING ___	11 TIRING ___	PPI_____ COMMENTS:
QUIVERING ___	EXHAUSTING ___	
PULSING ___	12 SICKENING ___	
THROBBING ___	SUFFOCATING ___	
BEATING ___	13 FEARFUL ___	
POUNDING ___	FRIGHTFUL ___	
2 JUMPING ___	TERRIFYING ___	
FLASHING ___	14 PUNISHING ___	
SHOOTING ___	GRUELLING ___	
3 PRICKING ___	CRUEL ___	
BORING ___	VICIOUS ___	
DRILLING ___	KILLING ___	
STABBING ___	15 WRETCHED ___	
LANCINATING ___	BLINDING ___	
4 SHARP ___	16 ANNOYING ___	
CUTTING ___	TROUBLESOME ___	
LACERATING ___	MISERABLE ___	CONSTANT___
5 PINCHING ___	INTENSE ___	PERIODIC___
PRESSING ___	UNBEARABLE ___	BRIEF___
GNAWING ___	17 SPREADING ___	
CRAMPING ___	RADIATING ___	
CRUSHING ___	PENETRATING ___	
6 TUGGING ___	PIERCING ___	
PULLING ___	18 TIGHT ___	
WRENCHING ___	NUMB ___	
7 HOT ___	DRAWING ___	
BURNING ___	SQUEEZING ___	
SCALDING ___	TEARING ___	
SEARING ___	19 COOL ___	

8 TINGLING ___	COLD ___	ACCOMPANYING SYMPTOMS:	SLEEP: GOOD ___	FOOD INTAKE: GOOD ___
ITCHY ___	FREEZING ___	NAUSEA ___	FITFUL ___	SOME ___
SMARTING ___	20 NAGGING ___	HEADACHE ___	CAN'T SLEEP ___	LITTLE ___
STINGING ___	NAUSEATING ___	DIZZINESS ___	COMMENTS:	NONE ___
9 DULL ___	AGONIZING ___	DROWSINESS ___		COMMENTS:
SORE ___	DREADFUL ___	CONSTIPATION ___		
HURTING ___	TORTURING ___	DIARRHEA ___		
ACHING ___	PPI	COMMENTS:	ACTIVITY:	COMMENTS:
HEAVY ___	0 No pain ___		GOOD ___	
10 TENDER ___	1 MILD ___		SOME ___	
TAUT ___	2 DISCOMFORTING ___		LITTLE ___	
RASPING ___	3 DISTRESSING ___		NONE ___	
SPLITTING ___	4 HORRIBLE ___			
	5 EXCRUCIATING ___			

Fig. 17–1. McGill-Melzack Pain Questionnaire. © R. Melzack, 1970.

This valuable tool provides sensory, affective, and evaluative measures of pain, with reliable and consistent results.

Quality

Patients use terms such as the following for different kinds of pain: "boring" pain of pancreatic carcinoma, "crushing" pain of angina, and "burning" pain of esophageal reflux. The McGill-Melzack Pain Questionnaire contains a useful list of descriptive sensory terms.

Variation

Pain can vary in many ways, but does so most commonly in relation to time, position, and activity. It can be present constantly or periodically, varying in frequency and severity at certain times of the day. Many patients find pain worse at night when fewer distractions occur. Certain pains are initiated or reduced by specific body positions. Pain can be affected by activities of daily living, such as breathing, eating, urinating, defecating, sitting, standing, or walking.

Response to Prior Therapy

Response to prior pain treatment provides useful information both for making a differential diagnosis and for planning strength, type, and timing of subsequent therapy.

SEVEN AIMS OF PAIN MANAGEMENT

If pain is due to a treatable problem that is unrelated to the primary disease process (e.g., toothache, local infection, or hemorrhoids), specific problem-oriented therapy should be given with analgesia. If pain is secondary to the primary disease but amenable to focal disease-oriented therapy (e.g., bone metastasis or nerve entrapment treatable by radiation therapy), such therapy should accompany symptom-oriented analgesia.

Identify the Cause

Medications should be given in adequate amounts and at appropriate intervals to relieve pain and to prevent its recurrence. Recurrent pain resulting from doses too small or given too far apart leads to dissatisfaction with the medication by the patient and often the caregiver. Such pharmacologically naive administration of analgesia often leads to a stepwise elevation of drug dose, resulting in increasing confusion,

disorientation, and sedation in the presence of unrelieved pain.

Prevent the Pain

Medications should be given routinely on a standing order basis, *not* as needed or prn. Additional analgesia required at certain times of the day or related
to certain activities may be provided on a prn basis,
preferably in anticipation of pain-inciting activity.

Patients should be awakened in the middle of the
night for their 4h dose of analgesic to prevent awak-
ening in the morning with recurrent pain. At 4h doses
of less than 30 mg of morphine or its equivalent, some
patients can increase their bedtime dose by 50 to 100%
and sleep for a full eight hours. This rarely succeeds
at higher doses. Pain prevention eliminates the fear
of recurrent pain, which itself can increase the analgesic requirement. Pain prevention also eliminates the
routine need for fast-acting analgesics (e.g., Demerol)
or for parenteral administration of standard analgesics. Rapid onset of analgesia is unnecessary when pain
remains adequately suppressed by standing oral or
rectal narcotic administration.

Erase the Pain Memory

Continued relief and prevention of pain help to
dissociate analgesic therapy from pain relief. This disruption of operant conditioning minimizes the potential
for psychologic dependence on the analgesic. Continued absence of pain itself may elevate the pain threshold and permit analgesic maintenance therapy at reduced doses.

Maintain Unclouded Sensorium

Narcotic-induced sedation usually occurs upon initiation or significant increase of narcotic therapy, but
typically is transitory (48–72 hours). Somnolence is
distressing to terminally ill patients and may itself
lower the pain threshold. Extreme somnolence, especially with constricted pupils and slowed respira-
tions, usually signifies excessive narcotic therapy or
progressive debilitation by the underlying disease
process. Rarely, pain may be so unresponsive that the
required narcotic dose causes significant sedation. Such
patients may benefit from concomitant administration
of a stimulant such as methylphenidate (Ritalin) 5–10

mg tid or dextroamphetamine (Dexedrine) 2.5–5 mg qd–bid.

Euphoria rarely occurs with appropriate narcotic therapy in terminally ill patients and is certainly *not* a goal of palliative care. *Loss of control* of one's emotional relationship with one's environment may lower one's pain threshold and thereby increase one's sense of pain.

Maintain Normal Affect

Most patients should be able to tolerate oral or rectal analgesia up until the last 12 to 48 hours before death. *Independence* and *increased mobility* gained from nonparenteral analgesia can elevate the pain threshold. For inpatients unable to take oral or rectal therapy, continuous IV infusion may provide more controlled, comfortable, and consistent analgesia than would repeated IM injections. Suppositories may allow families to maintain patients at home pain-free without need of IM injection or terminal hospitalization. Some families can be trained to give IM or SC injections when appropriate. Another recent option for home-care patients unable to swallow is continuous subcutaneous morphine by a battery-operated portable pump.

Provide Ease of Therapy Delivery

Side effects should be anticipated and prevented or minimized, so that relief of one symptom is not traded for the presence of another. All patients on narcotics become constipated and should be maintained on some form of bowel prep upon initiation of narcotic therapy (see page 220). Unchecked, constipation can be followed by obstipation and impaction, resulting in an acute abdomen requiring nasogastric suction, bowel rest, and/or surgery.

Prevent Physical Side Effects

Constipation

bowel prep protocol

Approximately 40% of patients on narcotic agents develop mild to moderate nausea, presumably from central apomorphine activity and peripheral decreased gastrointestinal motility. Some terminal patients have nausea even before initiation of narcotic therapy. Nausea associated with analgesic therapy hinders its efficacy. Prophylactic antinauseants are recommended for the first 48 hours of narcotic therapy. If nausea is

Nausea

BOWEL PREP PROTOCOL

Begin with a stool softener and gentle laxative:

a) dioctyl sodium sulfosuccinate 100 mg *plus* cas-anthranol 30 mg (Peri-Colace) 1 cap PO tid (range: 1 cap qd–2 caps tid)

b) dioctyl sodium sulfosuccinate 100 mg (Colace) 1 cap PO tid (range: 1 cap qd–2 caps tid) *plus* senna 187 mg (Senokot) 2 tabs PO hs (range: 2 tabs hs–2 tabs bid)

c) diocytl sodium sulfosuccinate 100 mg (Colace) 1 cap PO tid (range: 1 cap qd–2 caps tid) *plus* bisacodyl (Dulcolax) 5 mg PO hs (range: 5 mg PO hs–15 mg PO bid)

If no bowel movement in any 48-hour period add one of the following:

a) senna or bisacodyl as described above

b) Milk of Magnesia 30–60 ml PO hs (range: qd–bid)

c) lactulose (Chronulac 10 g/15 ml) 30 ml PO hs (range: 15–60 ml hs–bid)

If no bowel movement by 72 hours perform *rectal exam* to rule out impaction:

a) If *not impacted*, try *one* of the following:
  1) bisacodyl suppository, 10 mg PR
  2) magnesium citrate, 8 oz PO
  3) senna extract, 2½ oz PO
  4) mineral oil, 20–60 ml PO
  5) Fleet enema

b) If *impacted*:
  1) Disimpact manually if stool soft enough. (Consider pretreating patient with analgesic or tranquilizer.)
  2) Soften with glycerin suppository or olive oil retention enema, then disimpact manually.
  3) Follow up with enema(s) until clear and then increase intensity of daily bowel prep.

not a problem at that time, these agents may be tapered and then discontinued as tolerated. Occasionally, antinauseants cause clinically significant potentiation of analgesia and/or unwanted narcotic dose-limiting sedation.

prochlorperazine (Compazine) 5 mg PO q4h (range: 5 mg q6h–10 mg q4h)

If the above is too sedating or ineffective:
haloperidol (Haldol) 0.5 mg PO q8h (range: 0.5 mg q12h–1.0 mg q6h)

If sedation is desired in an agitated, nauseated patient:
chlorpromazine (Thorazine) 12.5 mg PO q4h (range: 12.5 mg q6h–25 mg q4h)

If gastric outlet obstruction is a problem, switch to or add to the above:
metoclopramide (Reglan) 10 mg PO q8h (range: 10 mg q8h–20 mg q6h)

recommended prophylactic antinauseants

Appropriately prescribed, narcotics rarely cause clinically significant respiratory depression. The threshold for such depression is always above the sedative threshold, which itself is above the analgesic threshold. With around-the clock narcotic administration, careful titration of dose for individual patients, and frequent reassessment, respiratory depression should not be a dose-limiting problem. Unexpected respiratory depression on stable analgesic dosage suggests metabolic derangement and /or central nervous system damage, requiring evaluation and treatment.

Respiratory Depression

Should analgesic-induced respiratory depression occur despite all due caution, it may be treated with naloxone (Narcan) 0.4–0.8 mg IV (IM or SC). Antagonist effects usually are immediate and may precipitate reemergence of suppressed pain or even a full-blown withdrawal reaction. One should remember that the half-life of one dose of naloxone is only 20 minutes, while the half-life of the excess narcotic agent may be several hours. Thus, repeated or even continuous drip naloxone administration may be required in severe cases of narcotic overdose.

Begin with the mildest analgesic and progress to strongest as needed. Each agent should be pushed to

ANALGESIA

Drug Selection and Escalation

its therapeutic/toxic limit before a stronger agent or a co-analgesic is applied. Initial doses and escalation increments should be individualized, with special attention to liver and kidney function.

Reassessment and Treatment Modification

Response should be assessed prior to each dose with attention to the extent and duration of pain relief following the previous dose. Once significant relief is obtained, that dose should be held for 4 to 5 half-lives of that agent to determine its full analgesic effect (e.g., morphine $t^1/_2 = 4h \times 5 = 20h$). At starting doses (5–15 mg morphine), a 50 to 100% increase in the standing dose in any 24-hour period usually is safe if required by the level of pain. At higher doses—for example, greater than 30 mg morphine—increases should be limited to 10 to 50% per 24h to fine-tune pain control and to avoid excessive adverse effects. Once adequate analgesia is obtained, patients with severe pain should be reassessed at least every 24 hours.

If severe pain breaks through the analgesia, a complete physical reevaluation is required to identify any reversible pain etiology or pain threshold-lowering problem, or to document any irreversible but prognostically important change in underlying disease.

Addiction

Psychologic dependence upon narcotics (addiction) is not a concern in terminally ill patients. Physical dependence upon narcotics occurs, but does not prevent reduction or discontinuation of narcotic therapy should the pain-inciting problem resolve (e.g., bone metastasis after successful radiation therapy).

Tolerance

Tolerance, leading to relentless escalation of narcotic dose, does not occur in terminally ill patients with pain. When controlled pain suddenly or progressively becomes more severe, primary causes (disease progression) and secondary causes (pain threshold decrease) are usually the explanation.

Brompton's Cocktail (Heroin)

The original Brompton's cocktail (solution) contained heroin, cocaine, chloroform water, and ethanol. Thorough studies have shown that heroin is no better than morphine in a Brompton mixture, and that a simple elixir of morphine in a flavored syrup vehicle is equally effective and no more sedating than a morphine Brompton cocktail. The amount of cocaine in the original Brompton's solution produced a slight increase in alertness and strength, but within two weeks patients became tolerant to these beneficial effects. The major reason for the continued used of heroin instead of morphine in Britain is its greater water solubility and its increased potency parenterally, which allows smaller injection volumes. However, the solubility and potency of hydromorphone (Dilaudid) allow for even smaller injected volumes, further obviating the need for heroin.

Most patients become unable to continue PO medication in their last 12–48 hours. When suppositories are unavailable or ineffective, morphine therapy should be continued SC or IM ($^1/_3$ to $^1/_2$ the PO dose) or IV ($^1/_4$ to $^1/_3$ the PO dose). In increasingly moribund and decreasingly communicative patients, pain cannot be readily assessed but should be assumed to be still present. Unless medically contraindicated, analgesic therapy should be maintained throughout the final hours to facilitate death that is free of physical pain. As cardiac output decreases, the dose interval may be extended to q6–8h.

Terminal Pain

Table 17–1 provides approximate oral and intramuscular dose equivalents for the narcotic analgesics most commonly used in this country. These doses vary among patients and should be used only as a guide to initiate or modify analgesic therapy. Of special note is the 3:1 intramuscular:oral dose equivalency for morphine, a distinct difference from the 6:1 equivalency stated in most pharmacology texts but well supported by British and Canadian hospice experience. In some patients, a 2:1 ratio has been observed. The subcutaneous dose is usually identical to the intramuscular dose. The intravenous dose, where applicable, is identical to or minimally lower than the IM dose and is associated with analgesia of somewhat earlier onset and shorter duration.

PHARMACOLOGIC THERAPY OF PAIN

Narcotic Dose Equivalents

TABLE 17–1.   Dose Equivalents for Control of Chronic Pain.[a]

Oral (PO) Dose (mg)	Analgesic[b]	Intramuscular (IM) Dose (mg)
150	meperidine (Demerol)[c]	50
100	codeine[c]	60
90	pentazocine (Talwin)[c]	30
15	**morphine**[d,e]	5
10	oxycodone (Percodan, Tylox)[e]	7.5
10	methadone[f]	5
10	diacetylmorphine (Heroin)	2.5
5	oxymorphone (Numorphan)[g]	1
4	hydromorphone (Dilaudid)[e]	2
2	levorphanol (Levo-Dromoran)	1

[a]**Equianalgesic doses** listed, obtained from a variety of sometimes conflicting studies, are meant only as guidelines for "by-the-clock," standing-order analgesic therapy of chronic pain. No analgesic listed is superior PO to its equianalgesic dose of PO morphine.
[b]**Dose interval:** Every 3–4h for all except the following: meperidine = q2–3h, levorphanol = q4–6h, methadone = q6–8h.
[c]Of little value in severe pain.
[d]Equianalgesic **intravenous (IV)** dose = 3–4 mg q3–4h.
[e]**Rectal suppositories** available or preparable. Per rectum (PR) dose equal to PO dose.
[f]**Caution:** Sedative side effects often accumulate despite inadequate analgesic effect.
[g]Available for nonparenteral use in rectal suppository form only.

The following chart shows gradations of pain and suggested analgesic regimens for each level.

RECOMMENDED ANALGESIC THERAPY

PAIN	ANALGESICS	FORMULATION	DOSAGE
Mild	aspirin	Tabs—325 mg Supp—325, 650 mg	
	or	Liquid—120 mg/15 ml	
	acetaminophen	Tabs—325 mg Supp—600 mg Liquid—120 mg/15 ml	650 mg q4h
Moderate	Aspirin #3 or	aspirin—325 mg codeine—30 mg	
	Tylenol # 3 or	acetaminophen—300 mg codeine—30 mg	2 tabs PO q4h
	Tylenol/codeine elixir	codeine—12 mg/5 ml acetaminophen—120 mg/5 ml	2 tbsp PO q4h
Severe	Percodan or	aspirin—325 mg oxycodone—5 mg	
	Percocet or	acetaminophen—325 mg oxycodone—5 mg	2 tabs PO q4h
	Tylox	acetaminophen—500 mg oxycodone—5 mg	

| Very severe | morphine elixir or | 15 mg/5 ml or more concentrated | 15–150 mg PO q4h |
| | hydromorphone (Dilaudid) | Tabs—1,2,3,4 mg Supp—3 mg Syrup—1 mg/5 ml | 4–40 mg PO q4h |

Aspirin is a preferred analgesic if inflammation is a major component of pain pathophysiology. Aspirin should be avoided in patients with a history of gastritis, ulcer, allergy to aspirin, chronic rhinitis, blood clotting dysfunction, or low platelet count. Concomitant use of antacids relieves some gastrointestinal symptoms but decreases aspirin absorption. Aspirin with meals often minimizes absorption interference. Arthritis and pain of bone metastases often respond to aspirin.

Mild Pain

A 60-mg dose of codeine is required for statistically significant increased analgesia over aspirin or acetaminophen alone. The use of high doses of codeine is limited because of its gastrointestinal and central nervous system side effects. Adverse side effects preclude the ability of most patients to tolerate doses over 60–90 mg PO q4h; a more potent narcotic agent should be used if pain remains uncontrolled at these doses of codeine.

Moderate Pain

Clinically, oxycodone is more tolerable than codeine and thus may be more effective at equianalgesic doses. One Tylox or Percodan may be preferable to aspirin or acetaminophen 650 mg plus codeine 60 mg, but should be supplemented with an additional 325 mg of aspirin or acetaminophen for optimal efficacy. Maximal Tylox dose is 2 tabs q4h due to acetaminophen content. Maximal Percodan or Percocet dose is 3 tabs q4h.

Severe Pain

Oral solutions of morphine usually contain 7.5 to 10% alcohol to extend the shelf life of the syrup vehicle. Chloroform water is substituted outside of the United States to avoid occasional gastrointestinal intolerance of alcohol/syrup mixtures. For patients not already on narcotics, 10–15 mg is a good starting dose. Doses for elderly, cachectic patients should be started at 2.5–5 mg. Patients on other narcotic agents should be con-

Very Severe Pain

verted to an equianalgesic dose of morphine, plus some additional amount based upon pain level and response to prior narcotic therapy. A steady-state body morphine level usually is attained in 16 to 20 hours (4 to 5 half-lives of morphine). If possible, dose escalation should be limited to two increases per day, for a total increment less than 50 to 100% of the starting dose in any 24-hour period. Once pain control is improved, subsequent titration should proceed more slowly, in 5–10 mg morphine-equivalent units per dose, no more than twice per day. This slow escalation should maintain a safe therapeutic level of morphine while minimizing unwanted sedation and respiratory depression. Some patients with rapidly progressive painful lesions, however, may require and tolerate more rapid and frequent dosage adjustments. Pain is controlled in over 80% of patients with a morphine dose less than or equal to 30 mg PO q4h. Although no absolute maximal dose exists, when patients require more than 150 mg morphine PO q3h, one should consider adding non-narcotic analgesic agents or completely reevaluating the patient in search of overlooked, treatable problems.

Intravenous Morphine Infusion   When inpatients can no longer tolerate PO or PR analgesia, constant, mechanically controlled IV infusion is often preferable to intermittent IM injections. A safe starting hourly dose is $^1/_4$ to $^1/_5$ that of the hourly PO dose. If a patient has gone without narcotics for more than 4 hours, the calculated hourly dose may be given IV push as a loading dose immediately prior to initiation of the constant infusion. Careful dose increases may be performed, as with PO dose escalation (no more than two escalations per day), usually by increments of 1–3 mg/h as tolerated. Both the increased IV potency and the usual concomitant poor metabolic activity of the patient requiring IV analgesia demand a cautious, gradual approach to adequate, safe levels of analgesia. The usual dose of IV morphine is 0.04–0.07 mg/kg/h (2.8–4.9 mg/h in a 70-kg adult), with a safe range of 0.5–200 mg/h.

Continuous Subcutaneous Morphine Infusion   When a patient's inability to tolerate PO analgesia is transient or when intravenous access is difficult or inappropriate, regular, four-hourly, subcutaneous injections of narcotic is an acceptable means of pain control. By switching from morphine to equianalgesic doses of the more soluble hydromorphone, the injection volumes can be reduced, thereby reducing the injection site discomfort. Recently, battery-powered compact portable pumps have been used to provide continuous subcutaneous analgesia. Patients or their families can be taught to insert a 25– or 27–gauge butterfly needle into subcutaneous tissue and to refill the pump syringe or bag-type reservoir on a daily basis. The subcutaneous dose is equal to the IM dose. A major limiting factor is the cost of the pumps ($200–$500), although some supply companies rent them at reasonable rates (which may be reimbursable by third-party payors).

Patients with neuroanatomically focal pain may benefit from intrathecal or epidural morphine administration. Connection of the appropriately positioned catheter to a subcutaneous Ommaya reservoir or battery-powered continuous infusion pump can provide excellent, constant local control with minimal systemic adverse effects. The reservoir or pump can be refilled regularly via subcutaneous injection of morphine solution by the patient or family. This arrangement may prove ideal for patients with local pain from vertebral body metastasis and nerve root compression. Pain control in these patients is difficult due to marked exacerbation of pain upon motion or weight-bearing.

Intrathecal/Epidural Morphine Administration

True allergy to morphine is rare. Patients may present with a local wheal-and-flare response or a disseminated rash, pruritus, and even bronchospasm. The only alternative noncross-reactive narcotics are meperidine (Demerol) and methadone, each of which has limitations in terminally ill patients (see following).

Morphine Allergy

Hydromorphone is essentially identical to morphine elixir at equianalgesic doses. Ambulatory patients often prefer the greater convenience of its pill form to the liquid morphine elixir. Multiple pill sizes allow easy titration. Further advantages of hydro-

Hydromorphone

morphone are its availability in rectal suppository form for patients unable to take oral medications and its high solubility, permitting small-volume parenteral injection.

Overwhelming
Pain

Additional pain control may be sought through adjunctive pharmacologic and anesthetic or neurosurgical approaches (see following). Whereas these measures may be used to reduce narcotic requirements in patients with lesser degrees of pain, they may be mandatory in conjunction with high doses of narcotic analgesics to establish adequate control of overwhelming pain. Through such intensive multidisciplinary therapy, pain control can be achieved in 95 to 99% of patients.

Other
Analgesic
Agents
Propoxyphene

Although no controlled clinical study has ever shown that propoxyphene is superior to placebo, it is often prescribed and has led to deaths due to overdose. *Propoxyphene has no role* in the management of chronic pain in patients with advanced disease.

Pentazocine

Pentazocine is a mixed narcotic agonist-antagonist. Although by weight it is almost equianalgesic with codeine, its use is severely limited by a high incidence of adverse reactions at therapeutic doses (sedation, drowsiness, confusion, blurred vision and hallucination, nausea and vomiting). Its PO absorption can be erratic, and it can cause local irritation at IM injection sites. Moreover, a shift from pure agonist narcotics to partial antagonists such as pentazocine or nalbuphine (Nubain) may cause narcotic withdrawal symptoms and reemergence of previously controlled pain. *Pentazocine should not be used in chronic pain control.*

Meperidine

Meperidine has little use in the management of chronic pain because of its short half-life of 2 to 3 hours. Repeated high doses at brief intervals to prevent pain recurrence have been associated with convulsions. Meperidine's potential inhibition of biliary sphincter spasm has not been clinically useful. Compared to other narcotics, it causes less pupillary constriction, thus reducing the opportunity to use this sign to monitor for dose excess. Meperidine given IM or SC may have some use in providing peaks of extra analgesia above a stable chronic narcotic for painful procedures (dressing change, disimpaction), or for ambulation in patients with pain only on weight-bearing (extensive bony metastases). Chronic use of PO meperidine may be attempted for patients with true allergies to morphine.

Levorphanol (Levo-Dromoran, tablets 2 mg) has *Levorphanol* the advantage of a longer half-life allowing q6h–8h dose intervals. Owing to its increased potency, however, it is usually easier to titrate initial narcotic therapy with hydromorphone (Dilaudid) or morphine elixir q4h and then switch to an equianalgesic dose of levorphanol: first q4h for 2–3 doses, then q6h for 1–2 days, then q8h if acceptable analgesia is maintained.

Methadone (tablets, 5–10 mg; elixir, 5 mg/5 ml) is *Methadone* a potent narcotic agent whose use is complicated by its peculiar pharmacokinetics. Methadone has a primary-phase half-life of 14.3 hours and a slower secondary-phase half-life of 54.8 hours in patients without prior methadone treatment. With repeated doses, a single half-life of 22.4 hours emerges. Equilibration and steady-state plasma levels occur 4 to 5 days after a new dose is begun. Unfortunately, there is little correlation between methadone plasma levels and analgesic efficacy. Clinically, methadone's analgesic effect lasts 3 to 5 hours. However, frequent dose escalations made at the usual intervals of every 4 to 6 hours can lead to methadone accumulation with toxic plasma levels even in the absence of adequate analgesia. Hepatic and renal dysfunction also increase its half-life. Concomitant use of agents that compete with methadone for plasma protein binding may elevate effective plasma methadone levels. Patients who are opiate-naive tend to have an exaggerated response to initial doses of methadone. The major indications for methadone, therefore, are limited to true allergy to morphine or to insurmountable difficulty in taking analgesics on a 4h basis. Another indication for gaining experience in the safe administration of methadone is that methadone costs considerably less than equianalgesic doses of morphine and hydromorphone. One effective approach to methadone therapy is to give a primary dose of 5 mg PO q6h for 48h. If pain is relieved, then continue at 5 mg PO q8h, extending intervals to q10–12h. If pain persists, then escalate the dose *slowly* and gradually once a day. The usual dose range for methadone is 40–80 mg/day. Once a desired level of analgesia is achieved, subsequent reduction of dose or prolongation of dosing interval should be limited to once every 3 to 4 days.

NON-PHARMACOLOGIC PAIN MANAGEMENT

Approximately 90 to 95% of patients with pain from advanced malignancy can be managed with pharmacologic measures alone. For the remaining 5 to 10%, the addition of palliative radiotherapy, surgery, anesthesia, or neurosurgery may provide pain relief unattainable by drugs alone or may be narcotic-sparing in patients with adequate pharmacologic control.

Palliative Radiation Therapy

Palliative radiotherapy can provide significant relief in patients with local pain-producing lesions, even in the face of advanced, disseminated malignancy (see Chapter 5).

Palliative Surgery

One is appropriately reluctant to subject terminally ill patients to further surgical procedures. Occasionally, however, surgery is the most appropriate or the only remedy for intractable pain. One week of surgical recovery may be justified by 3 months of predicted comfortable survival. Examples of appropriate palliative surgery are the following: incision and drainage of a tense abscess causing pain and spiking fevers; diverting enterostomy for painful intestinal obstruction; "toilet" mastectomy for patients with advanced, fungating breast masses; and bypass procedure for painful esophageal obstruction. Finally, palliative amputation or disarticulation of a painful, necrotic, ulcerated, infected limb relieves the patient of a tremendous metabolic and psychologic burden and provides pain relief. Palliative surgery requires careful consideration by the primary physician and a close working relationship with a skilled surgeon.

Biliary colic and even painful obstructive hepatomegaly can be relieved directly by transhepatic catheter insertion (see Chapter 2), obviating the need for surgery. Optimal care of pathologic fractures often requires internal fixations and/or prosthesis insertion. Aided greatly by newly developed glues, the orthopedic surgeon can reduce pain and minimize the immobility associated with such fractures. Prophylactic nailing of impending fractures (more than 50% of bony cortex destroyed on roentgenogram) can facilitate nursing care and prevent subsequent added disability.

Nitrous oxide-oxygen (50-50 mixture) sedation can provide safe, rapid-onset, short-acting, adjunctive analgesia for painful activities such as dressing changes, wound debridement, disimpaction, patient turning, and bed-to-chair transfer. Used most extensively by dentists, emergency room physicians, obstetricians, and obstetric midwives, portable nitrous oxide-oxygen systems now are used in inpatient hospices in Great Britain and Canada.

Palliative Anesthesia

General Anesthesia

Nerve blocks have long been used to relieve chronic pain and are covered in books and review articles. Approximately 5 to 10% of patients may benefit from such intervention. Nerve block techniques do have their own adverse effects and should be practiced only by an experienced anesthesiologist or neurosurgeon.

Local-Regional Anesthesia

The underlying principle in regional nerve block techniques is the differential sensitivity of sympathetic, sensory, and motor fibers to increasing concentrations of anesthetic or neurolytic agents. Careful neuroanatomic localization of the pain is prerequisite to consideration of nerve block techniques.

nerve block techniques

Once localized, the injection site is first infiltrated with increasing doses of local anesthesia, such as procaine, to document a positive effect. Only if pain relief is obtained consistently without significant adverse effects following 2 to 3 repeated anesthetic injections should a permanent block with alcohol or phenol be considered. Patients should be informed at the outset that not all blocks work and that, when they do, re-peated blocks may be necessary.

Some patients with local pain of long duration undergo a phenomenon of encephalization whereby pain becomes self-perpetuating at a central level. Nerve blocks are ineffective in such patients. Adverse side effects of sensory nerve blocks include unwanted sympathetic block (orthostatic hypotension, increased skin temperature, anhydrosis), diminished protective functional sensations (heat, proprioception, pressure), paresthesia, dysesthesia, urinary or fecal inconti-nence, and motor weakness or paralysis.

myofascial trigger point injections   Muscle imbalance following resectional surgery or radiation therapy, or associated with cachexia and bed rest, often results in pain from localized trigger points. Such pain is referred along a nondermatomal but re-producible patterned area. Periodic injection of local anesthetics into the trigger point may provide signif-icant palliative benefit.

somatic nerve blocks   Pain confined to a single nerve, nerve plexus, or nerve root dermatome often can best be treated with injections of local anesthetics. Once efficacy is safely demonstrated, neurolysis can be considered with al-cohol or phenol. Typical examples of pain in which somatic blocks may be beneficial are focal rib pain from soft tissue or bone metastasis, Pancoast superior sul-cus tumors, brachial plexus metastases, locally exten-sive rectal or pelvic carcinoma, head and neck tumors, and bladder spasm.

autonomic plexus blocks   Although the sympathetic system is not usually involved in the transmission of pain sensation, the pain of advanced malignancy may be relieved by plexus neurolysis alone or in conjunction with somatic block-ade. The most common examples are celiac plexus blockade for pancreatic cancer, stellate ganglion block-ade for burning pain in head and neck cancer, and stellate ganglion or sacral plexus blockade for painful tumor-induced reflex sympathetic dystrophy and pain-ful lymphedema following surgery for carcinoma of the breast or cervix. A major side effect of celiac plexus destruction is the loss of splanchnic vasoconstriction as an orthostatic compensation mechanism. Should this disabling effect not be alleviated by increased hydration, permanent neurolysis should be deferred.

Ablative or stimulatory neurosurgical procedures may obviate the need for repeated anesthetic blocks or provide pain control when all other techniques have failed. The neurosurgical approach to terminal patients usually is restricted to percutaneous procedures preceded by local anesthesia. Examples of ablative procedures include percutaneous rhizotomy and cordotomy, stereotactic ablations of sensory tracts within the midbrain, and stereotactic thalamatomy. Transnasal, transsphenoidal ablation of the pituitary gland (neuradrenolysis) also has provided relief of intractable pain, even in patients without endocrine-related malignancies.

Palliative Neurosurgery

Stimulatory neurosurgical procedures include peripheral nerve, dorsal cord, and deep brain stimulation. TENS (transcutaneous electrical nerve stimulation), a nonsurgical stimulatory technique, recently has been used in the management of pain in advanced malignancy. However, results have been mixed and benefits short-lived.

A variety of psychologic techniques show differing degrees of efficacy in patients with chronic pain. The use of these techniques with terminally ill patients has been limited, due to their dependence on the patient's motivation and power of concentration, and on the availability of trained therapists. Nevertheless, modalities such as hypnosis, relaxation therapy, and diversional therapy have no serious adverse effects and may be effective (see Chapter 6).

Psychotherapeutic Pain Management

Although most patients have received and failed standard chemotherapy, or are considered too ill to endure its adverse effects, single agent or combination chemo- or hormonal therapy occasionally can relieve symptoms of enlarging masses of advanced malignancy even when overall survival benefit is not expected. Such cancer-specific therapies also offer psychologic

Palliative Chemotherapy and Hormonal Therapy

support to patients and families who demand continuation of some disease-oriented therapy as long as possible (see Chapter 4).

The focal pain of a local bony metastatic lesion is usually best treated with analgesia and palliative radiotherapy, occasionally in conjunction with an orthopedic procedure. The pain of diffuse bony metastatic disease unresponsive to hormonal therapy or chemotherapy requires high levels of systemic analgesia. A large collective experience supports the use of nonsteroidal, anti-inflammatory, antiprostaglandin drugs (NSAID) as adjuncts to narcotic analgesia in such patients. NSAID therapy should be initiated with the best tolerated drug and should progress to more toxic agents only if pain remains unrelieved or if the potential narcotic dose-sparing effect is of maximum importance.

Adjunctive
Therapy
for
Relief
of
Bone
Pain

Recommended Anti-Prostaglandin NSAIDs:

ibuprofen (Motrin)	400	mg	PO q4–6h
zomepirac (Zomax)	100	mg	PO q4–6h

If the above are ineffective:

indomethacin (Indocin)	25–50	mg	PO q6–8h
aspirin	650–1000	mg	PO q4–6h
phenylbutazone (Butazolidin)	100–200	mg	PO q6–8h

Potential adverse effects of all NSAIDs are gastrointestinal distress, fluid retention, and platelet dysfunction, which contraindicate their use in thrombocytopenic patients and in those with bleeding disorders. Aspirin, indomethacin, and phenylbutazone are somewhat more ulcerogenic than ibuprofen and zomepirac. Phenylbutazone has significant potential for inducing bone marrow aplasia, especially when used for more than brief periods (1 to 2 weeks).

The bone pain of multiple myeloma does not respond well to NSAID, probably because bone destruction in this disease depends on osteoclast activating factor (OAF) rather than on prostaglandins. Perhaps the most difficult bone pain to manage is that of vertebral body metastasis, due to its exacerbation on weight-bearing. Analgesia adequate to permit painless movement is often excessive when the patient is supine. Severe cases may benefit from local intrathecal/ epidural morphine infusions (see earlier discussion). Alternatively, this type of patient may be one of the few for whom pre-activity intramuscular meperidine may supplement a standing, oral narcotic regimen.

The addition of moderately high-dose corticosteroids to narcotic analgesics often provides significant palliation of pain from compression of nerve roots or plexuses by tumor masses:

Nerve
Root
Compression
Pain

dexamethasone	4–8 mg	PO bid–tid
methylprednisolone	16–32 mg	PO bid–tid

The application of such adjuvant therapy (to relieve edema and swelling) should be considered when tumor masses entrap neuronal tissue in tight anatomic spaces, such as occurs in epidural metastases. Corticosteroids may help until further tumor expansion occurs.

High-dose corticosteroid therapy (following) usually controls headache and motor and sensory deficit with minimal or no narcotic supplement in patients with headache from primary or metastatic masses with associated intracranial edema:

Headache
from
Intracranial
Tumor

dexamethasone	8–25 mg	PO qid
methylprednisolone	32–100 mg	PO qid

Neurosurgeons have used up to 100 mg of dexamethasone per day with benefit to the patient. Whole brain radiotherapy, when appropriate, should be initiated as soon as possible. The corticosteroid dose should be maintained for 1 to 2 weeks after radiation to allow tumor response (see Chapter 5). The risk of peptic ulceration can be reduced with cimetidine (Tagamet) 300 mg PO qid and/or antacids between meals and at bedtime.

Painful distention of visceral organs and lymph nodes also may benefit from the same moderately high doses of corticosteroids used for nerve compression pain.

Visceral
Pain

Infiltration of soft tissues by tumor in nonclosed

spaces may also benefit from corticosteroid therapy. Lower doses usually are adequate:

dexamethasone	2–4 mg	PO bid–tid
methylprednisolone	8–16 mg	PO bid–tid

Secondary Infection   Tumor masses occasionally become secondarily infected by obstruction of normal drainage mechanisms or central necrosis. Topical debridement and antiseptic application may eliminate a large component of pain associated with such lesions. Systemic antibiotics may be useful in deeper lesions. Occasionally, palliative surgery, such as incision and drainage, may be required for optimal relief from a deep abscess.

Intestinal Colic from Obstruction   The severe, spasmodic pain of partial or complete obstruction can often be relieved with a combination of an antispasmodic and a stool softener:

diphenoxylate hydrochloride (2.5 mg) with atropine sulfate (0.025 mg) (Lomotil) 1–2 tabs PO q4–6h

or
loperamide hydrochloride(Imodium) 2 mg, 1–2 tabs PO q6h

plus
dioctyl sodium sulfosuccinate (Colace) 100 mg, 1 cap PO bid–qid

Combined with clear liquid diet and antinauseants, the aforementioned therapy can often obviate the need for nasogastric intubation and intravenous hydration, thereby allowing the patient to remain at home.

Lymphedema Pain   Moderately high-dose corticosteroids may be helpful in painful lymphedema. Jobst stockings or pneumatic pumping devices also may reduce pain, even in the absence of measurably reduced swelling.

Bladder Spasm Pain   Routine use of belladonna and opium (B & O) suppositories for severe bladder spasms from neurologic or infiltrative disease often obviates the need for systemic narcotic analgesia:

belladonna 15 mg, opium 30 mg (B & O No. 15A)   1 supp.
belladonna 15 mg, opium 60 mg (B & O No. 16A)   PR q4–6h

Chlorpromazine (Thorazine) 10–25 mg PO q4–6h may also be useful in bladder spasm or rectal tenesmus.

Neuromuscular Pain   Advanced malignancy, poor nutrition, and lingering effects of chemotherapy generally cause immunosuppression and therefore susceptibility to Herpes zoster (shingles) infection. Amitriptyline (Elavil) 25–150 mg PO hs is a useful adjunct to narcotic analgesia in these patients. Levodopa 100 mg and Benserazide 25 mg (Sinamet) 2 caps PO tid has also been reported to be effective.

Postherpetic
Neuralgia

Due to their sporadic, unpredictable, and often intense character, tics usually are not well controlled by constant-dose narcotic therapy. A variety of agents have been tried with variable success:

Intermittent
Stabbing
Pains
(Tics)

carbamazepine (Tegretol) 200–600 mg PO bid
(begin at 100 mg bid, increase by 100 mg/dose/day until pain relieved or maximum dose reached)
phenytoin sodium (Dilantin) 100 mg PO tid
(dose should be increased to achieve therapeutic blood level)
valproic acid (Depakene) 200 mg PO bid–tid

The most common cause for muscle spasm is an underlying or adjacent pain-producing process, such as a soft tissue mass or bone metastasis. Treatment with narcotic analgesics usually disrupts the pain-spasm cycle. Massage, physiotherapy, and heat also may be beneficial. If painful muscle spasm is not relieved, several agents may be tried. As a group they are limited by their sedative side effects, which may be problematic in patients already on high-dose narcotics.

Muscle
Spasm
Pain

diazepam (Valium) 2–10 mg PO q6–12h
baclofen (Lioresal) 5–20 mg PO tid
(increase by 5 mg per dose every 3 days as needed)
dantrolene sodium (Dantrium) 25–100 mg PO tid–qid
(increase by 25 mg per dose every 3 days as needed)

For severe, acute spasm:

diazepam (Valium) 2–10 mg IV/IM q6–12h
methocarbamol (Robaxin) 1000–3000 mg IM/IV q6–12h

Postamputation pain may be central or distal. Central pain requires systemic narcotic therapy. Distal pain often results from neuromata at the severed nerve endings and may best be treated with local anesthetic injections or neurolysis. Occasionally, distal pain may be relieved with application of transcutaneous electrical nerve stimulation (TENS).

Phantom
Limb
Pain

GASTROINTESTINAL
SYMPTOMS

Anorexia
Dehydration
Weight
Loss

Anorexia, dehydration, and weight loss are common, interrelated symptoms of most terminally ill patients (see also Chapters 2 and 11). Dehydration and weight loss usually are due to inadequate intake. Malabsorption, secondary to the underlying disease or its therapy, may play a role in patients with known abdominal disease. For most patients, however, anorexia is the major problem in maintaining nutrition and fluid balance. Careful, frequent administration of small amounts of favorite foods, food supplements, and fluids often prevents further progression of dehydration and weight loss. Intravenous and nasogastric feedings rarely are appropriate in the terminally ill.

Anorexia usually results from multiple etiologic factors. Disinterest in food is a common depressive symptom in patients who have lost the will to live. Usually, however, the anorexia of advanced disease includes actual physical difficulties with eating, such as unrelieved pain, mouth discomfort, dysphagia, nausea, constipation, and the lingering side effects of previous radiation therapy and chemotherapy. An uncontrolled malodorous ulcer also can decrease appetite, and hepatomegaly, abdominal tumors, or ascites can compress the stomach and thereby discourage adequate intake. Metabolic derangements and narcotic administration also cause nausea and decreased appetite.

The management of anorexia therefore depends on controlling all potentially reversible underlying etiologic factors. Nonspecific measures such as varying the menu and allowing patient selection; providing smaller meal portions; and serving meals in a room other than the patient's bedroom, with the patient getting dressed to eat, should be considered for all anorectic patients. Sherry or wine one-half hour before meals also may be useful. The only medications effective in directly stimulating appetite are corticosteroids, such as the following:

prednisone	10–20 mg	PO bid–tid
dexamethasone	2–4 mg	PO bid–tid

Anabolic steroids such as nandrolone phenpropionate (Deca-Durabolin) 200 mg IM weekly or fluoxy-mesterone (Halotestin) 5 mg PO tid have demon-strated anti-anorectic effects in some studies albeit with adverse side effects such as acne, masculinization, and fluid retention.

Cyproheptadine hydrochloride (Periactin) 4 mg PO tid 30 minutes before meals used to stimulate appetite produces variable results. Antidepressants and tran-quilizers may be effective when anorexia is primarily psychologic.

Mouth care is a frequently overlooked aspect of palliative care. Thirst is more often a symptom of poor oral hygiene than of actual dehydration. Monilial in-fections are common in terminally ill patients, espe-cially those on corticosteroids, broad spectrum anti-biotics, or chemotherapy. Tricyclic antidepressants, phenothiazines, antihistamines, anticholinergics, and local radiotherapy reduce saliva secretion and produce an uncomfortably dry mouth. Radiation and chemo-therapy also can cause painful mucositis. Mouth breathing and vitamin deficiency may contribute to oral pathology as well. Finally, weight loss can cause dentures to loosen painfully, and poor dental hygiene can lead to gingivitis, caries, and abscess.

Dry or Painful Mouth

Specific etiologies require specific remedies such as discontinuing offending medications and treating oral moniliasis if present. General measures begin with compulsive mouth care such as 2h mouth washing with equal parts of hydrogen peroxide, glycerine, mouth-wash (Cepacol), and saline. Once the mouth is clean, lemon glycerine swabs, ice chips, frequent sips of water, and sour candies are beneficial. Preventive den-tal hygiene and soft-relining of dentures should be per-formed regularly. Dietary supplementation with vi-tamin C (500 mg PO bid) and vitamin B complex may help in patients with significant malnutrition. Addi-tional useful agents include:

Dry Mouth:
carboxymethylcellulose (Xero-Lube, Sal-Eze) 5 ml PO prn
artificial saliva (Salivart) metered mist PO prn

Mouth Care Medications

Painful Mouth:

lidocaine (Xylocaine 2% viscous solution) 5-15 ml PO
  swish and swallow q3–4h prn (especially before meals)
dyclonine (Dyclone) 0.5%, 1.0%, 5–10 ml PO
  swish and swallow q4–6h prn

Monilial Infection (Thrush):

nystatin (Mycostatin Vaginal Suppositories) 1 supp. PO qid

clotrimazole (Gyne-Lotrimin Vaginal Suppositories) 1 supp. PO tid

ketoconazole (Nizoral) 200 mg 1 tab PO daily

Dysphagia   Dysphagia (difficulty with swallowing) and odyno-
phagia (pain on swallowing) often are extensions of
mouth care problems and therefore respond to similar
therapies. Esophageal lesions such as radiation-induced stricture or tumor mass compression are additional local etiologic factors. For the latter, palliative
radiotherapy, if feasible, is a useful approach. Nonspecific measures include pureed diets and the administration of medications in crushed or liquid form or
by rectal suppository. Aggressive local measures include nasogastric tube insertion or gastrostomy to ensure adequate nutrition. Parenteral hyperalimentation
rarely is indicated except in reversible transient dysphagia or when a few days of gained weight would
permit a patient to achieve an important goal. Specific
recommendations include:

Reflux Esophagitis:

antacids (Maalox Plus, Mylanta) 30–60 ml PO q2–4h
cimetidine (Tagamet) 300 mg PO q6h

Gastric Outlet Obstruction:

metoclopramide (Reglan) 10–20 mg PO q6–8h

Candidial Esophagitis:

ketoconazole (Nizoral) 200 mg 1–2 tabs PO daily
amphotericin B (Fungizone) 10–20 mg IV q12–24h × 5–7 days

Hiccoughs   Hiccoughs, involuntary contractions of the diaphragm, may be due to the following: toxic states such
as uremia; diaphragmatic or phrenic nerve irritation;
gastric distention; hepatic metastases; and intracranial
or medullary central nervous system tumors. Occasionally, pharyngeal stimulation (granulated sugar or
liquor) or CO_2 inhalation (direct administration or pa-
per bag rebreathing) may be effective. Simethicone
(contained in Mylicon, Mylanta, Maalox Plus) or nasogastric intubation also may be helpful in patients

with gastric distention. Drugs possibly of benefit because of their central nervous system effects are:

chlorpromazine (Thorazine) 25–50 mg PO/IM q4–6h
metoclopramide (Reglan) 10–20 mg PO/IM q6–8h
diazepam (Valium) 5–10 mg PO q4–6h

Dexamethasone (Decadron) 4–8 mg PO tid-qid may be of value in hiccoughs from diaphragmatic irritation secondary to metastatic hepatomegaly. Phenytoin (Dilantin) and carbamazepine (Tegretol) in full antiseizure doses may be useful in hiccoughs of CNS origin. Phrenic nerve blocks are rarely if ever needed in terminal patients.

Nausea and vomiting afflict 30 to 40% of terminal patients. Medications mentioned earlier as prophylactic antinauseants for narcotic analgesics form the backbone of drug management of symptomatic nausea and vomiting. Complete control, however, requires careful etiologic evaluation and, occasionally, the addition of antinauseant agents whose excessively sedating side effects preclude their use as routine prophylactic agents.

Nausea and vomiting can originate from central nervous system or alimentary tract alterations. Vagal stimulation by pharyngeal irritation, intractable coughing, gastric irritation, or gastric stasis can produce reflex nausea and vomiting unresponsive to antiemetics alone. Common causes of gastric irritation are corticosteroids, aspirin, nonsteroidal anti-inflammatory agents, alcohol, and blood. Gastric stasis may be due to the following: infiltration of the stomach by tumor, pyloric outlet obstruction by ulcer or tumor, diabetic autonomic dystrophy, narcotics, anticholinergics, or distal bowel obstruction. Specific treatment or bypass of regional problems is mandatory for adequate control of associated nausea and vomiting.

Nausea
and
Vomiting

Central nervous system nausea and vomiting may be emotional, mechanical, or chemical in origin. Pain, fear, and anxiety can cause nausea and vomiting that are best controlled by adequate pain management and psychosocial and psychopharmacologic therapy.

Raised intracranial pressure and vestibular stimulation from primary or metastatic brain tumors or carcinomatous meningitis can cause severe nausea and vomiting, requiring diagnosis and therapy as described in Chapters 3 and 5. Brain scan or lumbar puncture should be considered in patients with disseminated malignancy and intractable nausea and vomiting of uncertain origin.

Chemical stimuli reach the chemoreceptor trigger zone (CTZ) in the brain stem by way of the blood stream. CTZ stimulation causes activation of the vomiting center in the brain. Toxic states such as infection, radiation exposure, disseminated carcinoma, uremia, and hypercalcemia are all associated with CTZ stimulation. Narcotics, chemotherapy, estrogen, and digitalis are among the common medications that cause CTZ stimulation. Most antinauseants act directly on the CTZ and are most effective in treating nausea and vomiting of chemical origin.

Effective
Agents
for
Nausea
and
Vomiting

First Line Agents:
prochlorperazine (Compazine) 10 mg PO/IM, 25 mg PR q4–6h
haloperidol (Haldol) 0.5–2.0 mg PO/SC q6–8h
chlorpromazine (Thorazine) 12.5–25 mg PO/25–50 mg IM q4–6h
         50–100 mg PR q6–8h

Second Line Agents (Add to above):
metoclopramide (Reglan) 10–20 mg PO/IM q6–8h
cyclizine (Marezine) 25–50 mg PO q6–8h
dimenhydrinate (Dramamine) 50–100 mg PO/IM q4–6h
          100 mg PR q8–12h
pyridoxine 50 mg PO q6–8h
dexamethasone (Decadron) 4–8 mg PO bid–tid

Third Line Agents (Limited application):
tetrahydrocannabinol (THC) 10–20 mg PO q4–6h
methotrimeprazine (Levoprome) 5–10 mg PO/IM q6–8h
scopolamine 0.4–0.6 mg SC/IM q6–8h
atropine 0.4–0.6 mg SC/IM q6–8h

Management
of
Nausea
and
Vomiting

Management usually begins with administration of one of the first line agents listed above. At the same time, a search is begun to detect any reversible underlying etiology. Pharyngeal irritation from ulceration or tumor masses may require local anesthesia or even short-course radiation therapy. Intractable coughing spells may respond to increasing doses of narcotics. Gastric motility may be stimulated by metoclopramide (Reglan) 10–20 mg PO q6–8h. Medications that irritate the stomach should be discontinued if feasible. Constipation should be both treated and prevented. If intracranial pathology is found, dexamethasone (Decadron) 10–25 mg PO or IV q6h is helpful. Known CTZ stimulating medications should be discontinued if possible. If hypercalcemia is a contributing factor, it should be treated with corticosteroids, oral phosphosoda, or intravenous mithramycin.

Among the first line agents, prochlorperazine is most commonly used as initial therapy. Haloperidol and chlorpromazine are both effective although slightly more sedating than prochlorperazine. Among the second line agents, metoclopramide is most useful in gastric outlet obstruction, although it also has a direct effect on the CTZ. The antihistamines cyclizine and dimenhydrinate, although sedating, are useful when nausea has a vestibular component. These agents also suppress the vomiting center and may be useful additives to the first line agents. Pyridoxine is said to help in the nausea of pregnancy and may be useful in nausea secondary to abdominal radiotherapy. Dexamethasone has a general positive effect on some patients and may nonspecifically eliminate or minimize the sensation of nausea.

The third line agents have only limited application because of their significant side effects. Tetrahydrocannabinol has been shown in some studies to be more effective than prochlorperazine in chemotherapy-induced nausea. Major benefit was limited to patients under age 40 with previous positive experience with marijuana. Older patients experience extreme dysphoria and should not be given this agent.

Methotrimeprazine is a phenothiazine with significant analgesic and antinauseant effects. Because of its sedative properties it is reserved for use in bedridden patients when all other antinauseant measures have failed. If such patients are receiving narcotics, their narcotic dose should be reduced by 50% prior to initiation of methotrimeprazine. Methotrimeprazine is available only for injection in this country but is available in pill form in Great Britain (Veractil) and Canada

(Nozinan). Scopolamine or atropine is useful in moribund patients with intractable retching.

Constipation

Most terminally ill patients are constipated. The combination of inactivity, low residue diet, inadequate fluid intake, general weakness, analgesics, and tranquilizers results in infrequent bowel movements, causing both physical and mental distress. Hypercalcemia and hypokalemia further impair intestinal motility. Weakness and immobility causing fear of soiling may lead to voluntary fecal retention and subsequent constipation. Constipation causes fecal impaction, rectal bleeding, abdominal pain, and anorexia.

Management of Constipation

The management of constipation consists of both laxative administration and general normalizing measures. Correction of anorexia by increased food and fluid intake always should be attempted. Patients should be encouraged to add bran and fruit juices to their diets if tolerable. Increased activity—in particular, walking to the bathroom or using a bedside commode rather than a bedpan—is also beneficial. Ultimately, however, most patients will need laxatives and, as mentioned earlier, prevention is more effective than treatment.

Hydrophilic bulk-forming agents such as methylcellulose or mucilloids (Metamucil, Effersyllium) are somewhat unpalatable and depend upon adequate food intake and activity to be effective. These agents therefore are not useful. Similarly, stool softeners alone are rarely adequate to support regular defecation. Constipated patients should always be checked for impaction first and treated accordingly prior to initiation of oral laxative therapy (see Bowel Prep Protocol on page 220).

A common regimen for patients with significant constipation follows: dioctyl sodium sulfosuccinate 100 mg plus casanthranol 30 mg (Peri-Colace) 2 caps PO bid (or equivalent in liquid form), bisacodyl 5 mg (Dulcolax) 2–3 tabs PO bid, and lactulose 30 cc PO hs prn.

Patient education is crucial with laxative therapy to avoid swings from constipation to diarrhea. Patients must find their own optimal combinations for comfortable bowel function.

Although potentially the result of severe obstipation, significant bowel obstruction usually results from intestinal or gynecologic malignancies. Radiation and postoperative stricture and/or adhesions may also play a role. Similarly, chemotherapy with vinca alkaloids can produce paralytic ileus that may linger in debilitated patients. In advanced disease, the palliative goal is to manage bowel obstruction without resorting to nasogastric tubes or diverting surgery. *Bowel Obstruction*

The colicky pain of obstruction can be controlled by antiperistaltic agents such as: diphenoxylate with atropine (Lomotil) 2.5 mg, 1–2 tabs PO q4–6h, or loperamide (Imodium) 2.0 mg, 1–2 caps PO q4–6h. Small doses of codeine 15–30 mg PO q4h, morphine 5–10 mg q4h, or hydromorphone (Dilaudid) 1–4 mg q4h also may be useful. Unless the obstruction is high, oral medications are sufficient. With intractable vomiting or high obstruction, suppositories or subcutaneous injections may be required. In subtotal obstruction, stool softners dioctyl sodium sulfosuccinate (Colace) 100 mg PO tid should be administered along with small amounts of fluids as tolerated, to minimize the intraluminal component of the obstruction. Antiemetics—orally, rectally, or by injection—usually are necessary as well. High-dose corticosteroids (dexamethasone 8–10 mg PO tid–qid) are sometimes useful against obstruction due to peritoneal carcinomatosis, perhaps by reducing the surrounding inflammatory reaction and edema. *Management of Intestinal Obstruction*

Of the 5 to 10% of terminal patients with diarrhea, the most common etiology is overflow around fecal impaction. Management includes rectal examination, disimpaction, enemas, and improved bowel prep. Additional causes of diarrhea are bacterial or viral infection, radiotherapy-induced enteritis, malabsorption, broad spectrum antibiotics, tumor infiltration of colon or rectum, and anxiety. As always, specific etiologies require specific therapies such as antibiotics, pancreatic enzymes, or tranquilizers. Corticosteroid retention enemas or foams may reduce diarrhea that is secondary to infiltrating rectal carcinomas and may even decrease rectal discharge in such patients who have had palliative colostomies. Nonspecific therapies con- *Diarrhea* sist of chalk-containing compounds or anticholinergic agents for mild diarrhea, and narcotic antiperistaltic agents for the more typical moderate to severe diarrhea. Reduction of dietary residue also may be beneficial. Until the diarrhea is controlled, the perianal area should be protected with a barrier cream and frequent cleansing. Agents effective for diarrhea control are those described earlier for relief of colic from intestinal obstruction.

Ascites

Abdominal distention secondary to ascitic fluid accumulation may cause pain, anorexia, nausea, vomiting, and dyspnea. For management considerations see Chapter 2.

Stomal Care

Stomal therapy has become its own subspecialty with nurse clinicians and ostomy teams skilled in managing the physical and psychosocial problems of patients with ostomies. Family members should be encouraged to share in ostomy care as soon as possible. The addition of bismuth subgallate (Devrom) 500 mg PO tid–qid before meals or an appliance deodorant such as Banish 8–10 drops into the ostomy bag reduces odor at bag-changing time.

RESPIRATORY SYMPTOMS

Dyspnea

Dyspnea is a common and frightening symptom in terminally ill patients. Common etiologies include anemia, heart failure, pleural effusion, bronchospasm, bronchial plugging, pulmonary infection, pulmonary malignancy (primary or metastatic), chemotherapy- or radiotherapy-induced pulmonary damage, and underlying chronic obstructive pulmonary disease. In patients who experience the acute onset of dyspnea, cardiac arrhythmia, myocardial infarction, and pulmonary embolus must be considered. Traditional medical approaches to reversible etiologies should be applied (see Chapter 2).

Narcotics and tranquilizers are used to dissociate untreatable pulmonary pathology from the anxiety-provoking sense of air hunger. In the low doses described below and with careful monitoring of respiratory rate, these agents can provide remarkable relief for patients with moderate to severe hypoxemia, often obviating or reducing the need for supplemental oxygen:

morphine 5–15 mg PO q4h
hydromorphone (Dilaudid) 1–4 mg PO q4h
diazepam (Valium) 5–10 mg PO q6–8h
chlorpromazine (Thorazine) 12.5–25 mg PO q4–6h

As the inpatient's condition deteriorates, parenteral narcotics plus scopolamine (Hyoscine) 0.4–0.6 mg SC as a prn order for acute respiratory distress provide immediate comfort. Inhalation of an ultrasonically nebulized mist of bupivacaine (Marcaine) 2 ml (0.25%) with 2 ml of normal saline q4–6h has been used in England to anesthetize pulmonary stretch receptors and diminish the sense of dyspnea.

In the last 12 to 24 hours of life, patients with pulmonary pathology become too weak to clear large airway secretions, thus causing them to "rattle" when they breathe. Although the patient usually is comatose, the family needs to be reassured that the noisy breathing is not causing the patient distress. This disturbing manifestation can be alleviated by administering scopolamine or atropine as described for dyspnea to dry up excessive pulmonary secretions and relax the smooth muscles of the tracheobronchial tree. Scopolamine is usually preferred over atropine, because scopolamine depresses the central nervous system, whereas atropine stimulates it.

Persistent coughing can lead to insomnia, anorexia, nausea, vomiting, and pleuritic, musculoskeletal chest pain. Reversible causes such as bronchospasm, bronchitis, pneumonia, and pulmonary malignancies should be treated. General measures begin with removal of irritants, most commonly cigarette smoke. Humidified air and adequate oral hydration also are beneficial. Expectorants have no proven efficacy. Similarly, mucolytics are poorly tolerated and are rarely helpful. The mainstays of cough suppression are the following narcotic analgesics:

codeine 15–30 mg PO q4h
morphine 5–30 mg PO q4h
methadone 5–15 mg PO hs

Urinary retention increases the risk of bladder infection and, when severe, causes abdominal pain and renal failure. Most commonly, urinary retention in terminally ill patients is due to the following; bladder outlet obstruction (carcinoma of bladder, cervix, prostate, or benign prostatic hypertrophy, benign uretheral stricture); neurogenic bladder (epidural tumors compressing the spinal cord or cauda equina); and drugs (anticholinergics, sympathomimetics, tricyclic antidepressants). Patients with neurogenic bladders may benefit from bethanechol (Urecholine) 5–10 mg SC for acute retention and 10–30 mg PO tid–qid for chronic retention. Ultimately, most patients require indwelling Foley catheters (see following).

Urinary
Retention

Urinary
Frequency
and
Incontinence

Urinary frequency and incontinence are common problems in patients with advanced malignancy, causing physical and psychologic distress. Common causes of urinary frequency, aside from bladder dysfunction and obstruction, are: hypercalcemia, diabetes mellitus (primary or corticosteroid induced), and urinary tract infections. Urinary incontinence also may be the first sign of spinal cord compression by metastatic cancer.

Diabetes mellitus should be treated by reducing inciting factors or administering oral hypoglycemic agents or insulin. When associated with constipation and confusion, polyuria and polydipsia may be due to hypercalcemia. Urinary tract infections usually are accompanied by dysuria and cloudy or foul-smelling urine. Trimethoprim/sulfamethoxazole (Septra, Bactrim) 2 tabs PO bid is the preferred treatment because of its bid dosing. In sulfa-allergic patients, amoxicillin 250–500 mg PO tid is effective and well tolerated. Studies show that a single dose of 3 g of amoxicillin oral suspension is effective in 90% of patients with urinary tract infections, obviating the need for prolonged courses of therapy.

When urinary incontinence occurs only at night, a condom catheter may be sufficient. Chronic 24-hour use is seldom acceptable due to resultant maceration and inflammation of the glans penis. Therefore, indwelling Foley catheterization is the mainstay in the management of urinary frequency and incontinence as well as retention. Acidification of the urine with cranberry juice or ascorbic acid 1000 mg PO qid and administration of the urinary antiseptic methenamine hippurate (Hiprex) 1 g PO bid may reduce the incidence and severity of catheter-induced urinary tract infection. Methenamine is effective only if constant urinary acidification is maintained. Antibiotics should be used only when infection is symptomatic.

Regular bladder irrigation with sterile saline, dilute acetic acid, or bladder antiseptics may minimize sediment formation and infection. Effective antiseptic irrigants include citric acid and D-gluconic acid (Renacidin) 30–60 ml bid–tid or chlorhexidine (Hibitane) 1:5000 dilution in saline 100–200 ml daily. Silastic catheters, when available, are less susceptible to encrustation and clogging. Foley catheters should be changed routinely each month, whereas Silastic catheters may be left in place for 6 months. A two-day course of trimethoprim/sulfamethoxazole (Septra or Bactrim) 2 tabs PO bid should follow initial catheterization or catheter replacement immediately to reduce potential gram-negative sepsis.

Foley Catheter Maintenance

Pruritus (persistent, generalized itching) can be a troublesome symptom resulting in restlessness, anxiety, skin excoriation, and secondary infection. The most common causes in the terminal population are dry skin, obstructive jaundice, uremia, lymphomas, allergy, systemic drug toxicity, and superficial irritants or infections. Therapy begins with elimination of suspected allergens or irritants. A close-cut manicure reduces the risk of excoriation and secondary infection. Topical creams such as lanolin, alpha-Keri, crotamiton (Eurax), 1.0% hydrocortisone, triamcinolone 0.25% (Kenalog 1/4), or fluocinolone 0.01% (Synalar) applied tid or qid may be useful.

CUTANEOUS SYMPTOMS

Pruritus

Antihistamines:
chlorpheniramine (Chlor-Trimeton) 4 mg PO qid
hydroxyzine (Atarax) 25–50 mg PO q6–8h
diphenhydramine (Benadryl) 25–50 mg PO q6–8h
cyproheptadine (Periactin) 4 mg PO q6–8h

Anti-Pruritic Agents

Phenothiazines:
promethazine (Phenergan) 25 mg PO hs
trimeprazine (Temaril) 2.5 mg PO qid

Corticosteroids:
dexamethasone 0.75–2 mg PO bid–qid
prednisone 5–10 mg PO bid–qid

Anion Exchange Resin:
cholestyramine (Questran) 4 g PO qid

Tranquilizers:
diazepam (Valium) 2–10 mg PO q6–8h
chlordiazepoxide (Librium) 10 mg PO q8–12h

Antihistamines are effective in allergic conditions but carry significant side effects, including sedation and dry mouth. Chlorpheniramine and trimeprazine (a phenothiazine with antihistamine activity) tend to be the least sedative of the antipruritic agents. Periactin is a serotonin antagonist as well as an antihistamine and may work when other antihistamines fail. Low doses of corticosteroids may be required in some allergic or inflammatory conditions. Pruritus secondary to obstructive biliary disease or uremia often responds to cholestyramine (Questran), although the unpalatability of the powdered packets may limit its acceptance. Methyltestosterone 25 mg sublingually may be an effective alternative. Occasionally, pruritus is a symptom of anxiety and is therefore best relieved with tranquilizers.

Decubiti   Skin care of pressure-bearing areas in bedridden patients requires constant vigilance and expectant therapy. Deep bed sores are painful and difficult to heal in terminal patients with poor nutrition, weakness, and immobility. Therefore, the key to decubiti care is prevention (frequent position changes, egg-crate mattresses, sheepskins, and water beds). Simple camping air mattresses, half-filled with water, are inexpensive and useful. Most hospitals and nursing agencies have their own recipes for decubiti care which depend on the depth of the ischemic changes. Superficial dry lesions may respond to frequent gentle massage with skin creams. Superficial wet lesions should be dried by exposure to heat lamps or hair dryers and by application of unscented talc or magnesium and aluminum hydroxide (Maalox). Application of synthetic skin barriers such as Op-Site and Stomahesive reduces skin shearing, disperses pressure, and allows underlying superficial lesions to heal. These products usually are left in place for 3 to 7 days, thereby also reducing the amount of nursing care required.

Deep, ulcerated lesions require frequent cleansing and sterile redressing. An emulsion of 4% povidone-iodine solution (Betadine) with liquid paraffin in a 1:4 ratio is the favorite at St. Christopher's Hospice for cleansing and redressing ulcerated decubiti. Betadine ointment and Betadine viscous formula gauze pads used as dressings may substitute for Betadine solution or skin cleanser. Antibiotic impregnated gauze strips (Nu-Gauze) and Teflon-coated surgical dressings (Telfa) are also useful. To stimulate granulation tissue, the Palliative Care Service at the Royal Victoria Hospital recommends daily redressing with a turkish towel pad cut to the size of the decubitus, soaked in 20% benzoyl peroxide cream and packed into the ulcer under an occlusive dressing, protecting the surrounding skin with petroleum jelly. Granulex, an aerosol solution of trypsin, balsam peru, and castor oil, applied twice a day is also an effective granulation tissue stimulant. Judicious use of collagenase (Santyl) or dextranomer (Debrisan) may be helpful in ulcers with copious necrotic debris. Surgical debridement may be required in severe cases. Topical antibiotics should be avoided due to the high risk of allergic sensitization or the development of resistant bacterial infections. Systemic antibiotics are indicated only in the presence of spreading cellulitis. Dietary supplementation with vitamin C 500 mg PO bid and vitamin A 25,000 units daily may aid tissue healing.

Care of Deep Cutaneous Ulcers

Fungating malignant lesions can produce pain, nausea, anorexia, and psychologic distress because of their appearance and odor. Specific chemotherapy, palliative radiotherapy, and palliative surgery should be offered when appropriate. Nonspecific measures are similar to those used in the management of deep decubiti. An oxidizing solution such as dilute Dakin's

Fungating Growths

solution may be useful in early debridement but should be discontinued when the lesion is free of necrotic debris to allow for adequate granulation. Systemic antibiotics may be beneficial if signs of local sepsis are present. If anaerobes are expected, metronidazole (Flagyl) 500 mg PO tid may be beneficial. Gauze soaked in epinephrine (1:1000) can be applied to open lesions to reduce capillary bleeding. Vulvar lesions may respond to frequent cleansing with chlorhexidine gluconate (Hibiclens). Room deodorizers should be used as needed.

CENTRAL NERVOUS SYSTEM SYMPTOMS

Weakness

Considered a prelude to helplessness, dependency, and impending death, progressive weakness provokes both anxiety and depression. Many factors contribute to weakness; some, such as fever or anemia, are amenable to specific therapy. In this setting, physical therapy is aimed more at stabilization than rehabilitation, although a resultant change in the patient's underlying attitude can help. As disability increases, assistance should be offered judiciously to avoid overwhelming the patient with manifest evidence of increasing physical dependency. Improved nutrition will help reverse or stabilize generalized weakness; the mood-elevating and appetite-stimulating effects of corticosteroids may be beneficial. The anticatabolic effects of androgen therapy—nandrolone phenpropionate (Deca-Durabolin) 200 mg IM q week, or fluoxymesterone (Halotestin) 5 mg PO tid—may also be helpful. Patients with weakness in addition to lethargy may benefit from a nonspecific stimulant such as methylphenidate (Ritalin) 5–10 mg PO tid.

Regional Weakness

Regional weakness or paralysis usually is secondary to neuroanatomic lesions in the brain, spinal cord, or peripheral nerves. Intracranial lesions and nerve compression syndrome may respond to high-dose corticosteroids (dexamethasone 8–25 mg PO qid). Peripheral neuropathy from chemotherapeutic agents such as vincristine or hexamethylmelamine may improve with pharmacologic doses of pyridoxine (vitamine B_6) 100 mg PO tid. Physical medicine can provide supportive appliances, exercises to reduce painful spasticity, and limb retraining. The palliative approach to focal loss of function aims to minimize further dysfunction, maximize remaining function, and support a positive patient attitude—not an easy task.

Reactive depression is an appropriate response to progressive disease and impending death. With skilled control of physical symptoms and psychosocial support from families and friends, patients can face their illness with remarkable courage and resolve. The most effective management of depression is time. Time is required to allow the patient and family to deal with the emotional and spiritual aspects of their impending loss. Nevertheless, a subset of patients with deep, persistent despair and symptoms of insomnia, anorexia, and emotional lability may benefit from tricyclic antidepressants.

Depression

amitriptyline (Elavil) 25–150 mg PO hs
imipramine (Tofranil) 50–150 mg PO hs
doxepin (Sinequan) 50–150 mg PO hs

Antidepressants

Administered as a single bedtime medication, the antidepressant's sedative side effects are used to advantage in combating insomnia. The nightly dose should begin at the 25–50 mg range and then increase by 25–50 mg every 2 to 3 days as tolerated. Clinically detectable antidepressive effects do not appear until 2 to 4 weeks after the start of therapy. Elderly or cachectic patients may need or tolerate only 100 mg as a maximal maintenance dose. Patients with agitated depression may benefit from a more even distribution of the sedative effect of the antidepressant agents by taking them in divided doses throughout the day, such as 50 mg PO tid. Troublesome potential side effects are confusion, constipation, and dry mouth. Monoamine-oxidase inhibitors should be avoided due to their many adverse interactions with dietary substances and medications. Electroconvulsive therapy has no place in the therapy of terminally ill patients.

Anxiety is similar to depression in its responsiveness to time and attention. Dyspneic patients tend to be the most anxious but obtain remarkable relief from

Anxiety

small doses of morphine and occasionally benzodiazepines. Phenothiazines and benzodiazepines are useful
tranquilizers for anxious patients. Phenothiazines are
preferable in anxious patients who are also on narcotic
agents for pain or who are suffering from nausea or
pain of rectal or bladder spasm. Patients receiving
prochlorperazine (Compazine) for antiemesis can obtain relief of both anxiety and nausea with chlorpromazine (Thorazine) instead. Benzodiazepines are effective anxiolytics and muscle relaxants. Due to their
prolonged half-life ($t^1/_2$), frequent administration may
lead to accumulation of drug and consequent intoler-
able dullness, incoordination, confusion, or sedation,
especially in the elderly. Diazepam (Valium, $t^1/_2$ =
25–65h) often can be given only at bedtime with full
anxiolytic effect throughout the day and accumulation
problems occurring only after several weeks, if at all.
Transient reactive anxiety may be treated with lorazepam (Ativan, $t^1/_2$ = 10–15h) or oxazepam (Serax,
$t^1/_2$ = 5–10h), although in acute anxiety states, diaze-
(Valium) has the most rapid oral absorption. Intramuscular Valium has an unpredictable absorption and
should not be used to treat anxiety. Chlordiazepoxide
(Librium) has a $t^1/_2$ of 5–30h. Benzodiazepines tend to
have a general depressive effect and should be reserved for anxiety unresponsive to psychosocial support or to low-dose phenothiazines. Chronic use of benzodiazepines also can lead to physical dependence with
significant withdrawal symptoms occurring upon ab-
rupt discontinuation.

Anxiolytics

Phenothiazines:
chlorpromazine (Thorazine) 10–50 mg PO tid
                          or
                          12.5–25 mg PO q4h
                          with narcotics
promazine (Sparine) 25–50 mg PO tid

Benzodiazepines:
diazepam (Valium) 2.5–10 mg PO tid–qid
chlordiazepoxide (Librium) 5–20 mg PO tid–qid
lorazepam (Ativan) 1–3 mg PO bid–tid
oxazepam (Serax) 5–15 mg PO tid–qid

Insomnia

Inability to fall asleep or to remain asleep for an
adequate rest period usually is secondary to unrelieved

physical or mental distress. Even after physical pain is controlled with appropriate 4h analgesia, prolonged bed rest or diminished diversion during the late night hours may lead to sleep-depriving night pain. In such patients, an additional 5–10 mg of morphine or its equivalent is the most effective hypnotic. Night sweats also can interrupt needed sleep and may respond well to indomethacin (Indocin) 100 mg suppository PR hs or 25–50 mg PO hs. As mentioned earlier, insomnia can be a symptom of depression or anxiety and is thus best treated by bedtime administration of appropriate antidepressants or anxiolytics. Patients with insomnia who are already on chlorpromazine (Thorazine) may benefit from a double dose of chlorpromazine at bedtime. The confusion and disorientation of organic brain syndrome respond well to haloperidol (Haldol) 1–5 mg PO hs with daytime supplements to relieve agitation. Insomnia in some patients may stem from a fear of sleep, symbolic of loss of control, or fear of not waking up. Increased counseling and reassurance is useful.

A general hypnotic agent can relieve simple insomnia. Barbiturates and long-acting benzodiazepines should be avoided due to their long half-lives. Chloral hydrate, prepared in capsule and liquid form, is one of the best hypnotics available in the United States. Short-acting benzodiazepines may be adequate for sleep induction, obviating the problem of cumulative sedation. Unfortunately, all benzodiazepines suppress stages 3 and 4 of the sleep cycle and may cause nightmares. Flurazepam (Dalmane $t^{1/2} = 50$–250h) 15–30 mg PO hs is an effective hypnotic but frequently causes morning hangovers and should be used only as a last resort. Chlormethiazole (Heminevrin) 500–1000 mg PO hs is an effective British nonbenzodiazepine hypnotic especially useful in the elderly but unavailable in the United States. In selected patients, 30–60 ml of brandy may be adequate.

chloral hydrate	500–1500 mg	PO hs	*Hypnotics*
promethazine (Phenergan)	25–50 mg	PO hs	
chlorpromazine (Thorazine)	50–100 mg	PO hs	
amitriptyline (Elavil)	25–150 mg	PO hs	

oxazepam (Serax)	10–30 mg	PO hs
lorazepam (Ativan)	2–4 mg	PO hs
diazepam (Valium)	5–15 mg	PO hs

Confusion

Common, occasionally reversible toxic and metabolic etiologies of confusion include the following: drugs (tranquilizers, hypnotics, antidepressants, alcohol, analgesics), uremia, hypoglycemia, hypercalcemia, hyponatremia, hypomagnesemia, hypoxia, hypercapnia, sepsis, pneumonia, tertiary syphilis, postictal states, and intracranial malignancy. Cerebral atrophy secondary to chronic ethanol abuse or cerebral arteriosclerosis also may contribute to confusion or dementia by increasing susceptibility to the physical and even psychologic causes of confusion. The most common psychologic factor leading to confusion is an altered, unfamiliar environment, especially for elderly patients. Familiar faces, voices, and objects; large readable room clocks and calendars; and increased attention from staff can help maintain orientation.

Reversible toxic and metabolic problems should be corrected. Supplemental oxygen can produce dramatic effects in hypoxemic patients, even if they are not clinically dyspneic. High-dose corticosteroids (dexamethasone 10–25 mg PO qid) can reverse obtundation secondary to intracranial malignancy in days. Note that some confused patients are not distressed by their confusion and remain pleasantly quiet and content. Such patients do not require psychotropic therapy. Most patients, however, are restless, frustrated, and distressed by confusion. Moreover, their behavioral responses strain and negatively influence their interactions with health care staff and families. Such patients require sedation with major tranquilizers. Occasionally, patients may be able to reorganize their thinking with treatment; most become quieter and more tractable, but remain confused.

Major Tranquilizers for Confusion or Agitation

haloperidol (Haldol) 5–10 mg IM q2h for acute agitation
                        0.5–5 mg PO q6–12h for chronic confusion
trifluoperazine (Stelazine) 2–5 mg PO q8–12h
thioridazine (Mellaril) 50–100 mg PO hs or 25 mg PO tid
chlorpromazine (Thorazine) 25–50 mg PO q6–8h

Haloperidol (Haldol) is the least sedative of the

aforementioned agents, but has the highest risk of tardive dyskinesia. Benztropine mesylate (Cogentin) 1–4 mg PO q12–24h may be needed in patients showing tremors or rigidity. Patients with mild organic brain syndrome usually respond well to haloperidol 0.5–1 mg PO q am, 1–2 mg PO hs. Trifluoperazine (Stelazine) has fewer parkinsonian side effects than haloperidol, but carries greater cardiovascular risks (arrhythmia, hypotension). Thioridazine (Mellaril) and chlorpromazine (Thorazine) are most useful when extra sedation is required.

Fitful thrashing and restlessness during the last 12–24 hours of life may result from persistent unrelieved physical symptoms such as pain. Agitation may be the patient's only means of communicating distress. Even in the absence of pain, the treatment of choice for such patients is parenteral analgesics. In patients already on narcotic agents, narcotics should be continued with *gradual* increase in dosage and reduction in dosing intervals from q6 to q4h to maintain tranquility without abruptly suppressing respiration. In patients not already on narcotics, morphine 2.5–5 mg SC q4h or hydromorphone (Dilaudid) 1–2 mg SC q4h are reasonable starting doses. Supplemental sedation with haloperidol (Haldol) 1–2 mg SC q2–4h also may be beneficial, but should not be given without some analgesia to assure relief of any persisting terminal pain. Sporadic muscle twitching, unsuppressed by analgesics or haloperidol, may respond to diazepam (Valium) 5–10 mg IV/IM q6h–8h. The use of scopolamine or atropine for terminal airway secretions ("death rattles") has been discussed.

Terminal Restlessness

Patients with primary or secondary brain malignancies present with or are at a high risk for seizures. Phenytoin (Dilantin) remains the drug of choice despite its multiple drug interactions and adverse side effects. Phenytoin is available in liquid or capsule form and must be used in amounts adequate to maintain therapeutic blood levels to suppress and prevent seizures. Therapy begins with a loading dose of 1 g of phenytoin in divided doses over the first 24 hours,

Seizures

followed by maintenance of 300–600 mg daily with adjustments based on drug levels. Although high-dose corticosteroids suppress many symptoms of intracranial malignancy, they also alter the metabolism of phenytoin so that 300 mg per day may be inadequate. Breakthrough seizures in the face of therapeutic blood levels of phenytoin may be suppressed by the addition of carbamazepine (Tegretol) 200–600 mg PO q8–12h, valproic acid (Depakene) 15–30 mg/kg/day, or phenobarbital 30–60 mg PO q6–8h. Aside from causing considerable sedation, phenobarbital is the best tolerated second line anticonvulsant.

Status epilepticus is a rare but distressing occurrence in terminal patients. Airway maintenance, tongue protection, and intravenous diazepam (Valium) 5–10 mg as needed are the usual initial maneuvers. In previously untreated patients, phenytoin (Dilantin) loading may be accomplished by slow IV push (500 mg over 10 minutes, then 250 mg over 5 minutes q2h × 2). Diazepam's effect tends to be transient (5–20 minutes), and IV or IM phenobarbital may be needed. In patients previously on phenytoin whose blood level of drug is uncertain, an additional 400–500 mg of intravenous phenytoin may be given. Should phenobarbital be needed, a loading dose of 120–240 mg can be given slowly IV at a rate of 25 mg per minute, watching for respiratory depression and hypotension in patients previously treated with diazepam. Repeated doses may be given every 15–20 minutes, rarely exceeding a total of 400–600 mg in the first 2h. A maintenance dose of 1–5 mg phenobarbital/kg body weight/day can be given as continuous IV infusion, intermittent q6h IV infusion, or intermittent IM injection.

Patients with seizures who are unable to swallow in their terminal 12–24 hours usually can be maintained on IM phenobarbital alone 1–5 mg/kg/day in divided doses. If this is inadequate, supplemental IV diazepam, IV phenytoin, or nasogastrically administered phenytoin may be needed.

CATASTROPHIC EMERGENCIES   Panic is the major problem when catastrophic emergencies occur in terminally ill patients. Appropriate management, therefore, is prevention and contingency planning. For example, if sudden external bleeding is anticipated, abundant absorbent pads, towels, and blankets should be on hand to contain the bleeding and minimize psychologic trauma to the aware patient, the observing family, or the inpatient roommate.

Major hemorrhage from any site, pulmonary embolus, myocardial infarction, a severe choking attack, or a fracture of a long bone are best treated by an immediate intramuscular (or intravenous, if an IV line is in place) injection of morphine 10–20 mg or hydromorphone (Dilaudid) 3-6 mg plus scopolamine (Hyoscine) 0.4-0.6 mg. This combination has the added advantage of inducing retrograde amnesia for the catastrophic event should the patient recover.

For a more general analysis of the factors involved in the etiology and management of the symptoms and problems in terminally ill patients, the reader is refered to the relevant chapters in this volume.

SELECTED READING

General

1. Ajemian, I., and Mount, B.M. (Eds.): The R.V.H. Manual on Palliative/Hospice Care. New York, Arno Press, 1980.
2. Freitag, J.J., and Miller, L.W.: Manual of Medical Therapeutics. Boston, Little, Brown and Co., 1980.
3. Saunders, C.M. (Ed.): The Management of Terminal Disease. Chicago, Year Book Medical Publishers, 1978.
4. Twycross, R.G., and Ventafridda, V. (Eds.): The Continuing Care of Terminal Cancer Patients. Oxford, Pergamon Press, 1980.

Pain

1. Barber, J., and Gitelson, J.: Cancer pain: psychological management using hypnosis. CA-Cancer J. Clinicians, 30:130–136, 1980.
2. Black, P.M.: Management of cancer pain: an overview. Neurosurgery, 5:507–518, 1979.
3. Bonica, J.J., and Ventafridda, V. (Eds.): Advances in Pain Research and Therapy. New York, Raven Press, 1979.
4. Brechner, V.L., Ferrer-Brechner, T., and Allen, G.D.: Anesthetic measures

in management of pain associated with malignancy. Semin. Oncol., 4:99–108, 1977.

5. Ettinger, D.S., Vitale, P.J., and Trump, D.L.: Important clinical pharmacologic considerations in the use of methadone in cancer patients. Cancer Treat. Rep., 63:457–459, 1979.

6. Graham, C., Bond, S.S., Gerkovich, M.M., and Cook, M.R.: Use of the McGill Pain Questionnaire with assessment of cancer pain: replicability and consistency. Pain, 8:377–387, 1980.

7. Griffin, G.C., Campbell, V.D., and Jones, R.: Nitrous oxide-oxygen sedation for minor surgery. J.A.M.A., 245:2411–2413, 1981.

8. Kaiko, R.F., et al.: Analgesic and mood effects of heroin and morphine in cancer patients with postoperative pain. N. Engl. J. Med., 304:1501–1505, 1981.

9. Kernbaum, S., and Hauchecome, J.: Administration of Levodopa for relief of Herpes Zoster pain. J.A.M.A., 246:132–134, 1981.

10. Long, D.M.: Surgical therapy of chronic pain. Neurosurgery, 6:317–328, 1980.

11. Maxwell, M.B.: How to use methadone for the cancer patient's pain. Am. J. Nurs., 80:1606–1609, 1980.

12. McCaffery, M.: How to relieve your patients pain fast and effectively with oral analgesics. Nurs., 10:58–63, 1980.

13. McCaffery, M.: Relieving pain with noninvasive techniques. Nurs., 12:55–57, 1980.

14. Melzack, R.: The McGill Pain Questionnaire: major properties and scoring methods. Pain, 1:277–299, 1975.

15. Melzak, R., Mount, B.M., and Gordon, J.M.: The Brompton mixture versus morphine solution given orally: effects on pain. C.M.A.J., 120:435–438, 1979.

16. Merritt, J.L.: Management of spasticity in spinal cord injury. Mayo. Clin. Proc., 56:614–622, 1981.

17. Minow, R., Janis, M., and Posner, L.: Continuous subcutaneous infusion of morphine in the cancer patient. Proc. Am. Soc. Clin. Oncol., 22:397, 1981.

18. Miser, A.W., Miser, J.S., and Clark, B.S.: Continuous intravenous infusion of morphine sulfate for control of severe pain in children with terminal malignancy. J. Pediatr., 96:930–932, 1980.

19. Moertel, C.G., Ahmann, D.L., Taylor, W.F., and Schwartau, N.: Relief of pain by oral medication: A controlled evaluation of analgesic combinations. J.A.M.A., 241:2408–2412, 1974.

20. Mount, B.M., Melzak, R., and Mackinnon, K.H.: The management of intractable pain in patients with advanced malignant disease. J. Urol., 120:720–725, 1978.

21. Onofrio, B.M., Yaksh, T.L., and Arnold, P.G.: Continuous low-dose intrathecal morphine administration in the treatment of chronic pain of malignant origin. Mayo Clin. Proc., 56:516–520, 1981.

22. Perret, G., and McDonnell, D.: Neurosurgical control of pain in the patient with cancer. Curr. Probl. Cancer, 1:1–27, 1977.

23. Pilon, R.N., and Baker, A.R.: Chronic pain control by means of an epidural catheter. Cancer, 37:903–905, 1976.

24. Pollen, J.J., and Schmidt, J.D.: Bone pain in metastatic cancer of the prostate. Urology, 13:129–134, 1979.

25. Rutter, P.C., Murphy, F., and Dudley, H.A.F.: Morphine: controlled trial of different methods of administration for postoperative pain relief. Br. Med. J., 1:12–13, 1980.

26. Shumacker, H.B.: Management of moderate lymphedema. Arch. Surg., 116:1097–1098, 1981.

27. Twycross, R.G.: Clinical experiences with diamorphine in advanced malignant disease. Int. J. Clin. Pharmacol., *9*:184–198, 1974.
28. Twycross, R.G.: The measurement of pain in terminal carcinoma. J. Int. Med. Res., *4*(Suppl 2):58–67, 1976.
29. Zeissler, R., Rose, G.B., and Nelson, P.A.: Postmastectomy lymphedema: late results of treatment in 385 patients. Arch. Phys. Med. Rehabil., *53*:159–166, 1972.

Gastrointestinal Symptoms

1. Abramowicz, M. (Ed.): Ketoconazole (Nizoral). A new antifungal agent. Med. Lett. Drugs Ther., *23*:85–87, 1981.
2. Ginsburg, C.H., Barden, G.L., Tauber, A.I., and Trier, J.S.: Oral Clotrimazole in the treatment of esophageal candidiasis. Am. J. Med., *71*:891–895, 1981.
3. Mazzaferri, E.L., O'Dorisio, T.M., and LoBuglio, A.F.: Treatment of hypercalcemia associated with malignancy. Semin. Oncol., *5*:141–153, 1978.
4. Poster, D.S., Penta, J.S., Bruno, S., and MacDonald, J.S.: Tetrahydrocannabinol in clinical oncology. J.A.M.A., *245*:2047–2051, 1981.
5. Sanders, J.F.: Lactulose syrup assessed in a double-blind study of elderly constipated patients. J. Am. Geriatr. Soc., *26*:236–239, 1978.
6. Schulze-Delrieu, K.: Drug therapy: metaclopramide. N. Engl. J. Med., *305*:28–33, 1981.
7. Seigel, L.J., and Longo, D.L.: The control of chemotherapy-induced emesis. Ann. Intern. Med., *95*:352–359, 1981.
8. Straus, A.K., Roseman, D.L., and Shapiro, T.M.: Peritoneovenous shunting in the management of malignant ascites. Arch. Surg., *114*:489–491, 1979.

Urinary Symptoms

1. Abramowicz, M. (Ed.): Treatment of urinary tract infections. Med. Lett. Drugs Ther., *23*:69–70, 1981.

Cutaneous Symptoms

1. Ahmed, M.C.: Choosing the best method to manage pressure ulcers. Nurs. Drug Alert, *4*:113–120, 1980.
2. Foltz, A.T.: Nursing care of ulcerating metastatic lesions. Oncol. Nurs. for 1980; *7*:8–13.
3. Millikan, L.E.: Topical corticosteroid therapy. Miss. Med., *78*:237–242, 1981.
4. Rao, D.B., Sane, P.G., and Georgiev, E.L.: Collagenase in the treatment of dermal and decubitus ulcers. J. Am. Geriatr. Soc., *23*:22–30, 1975.
5. Reuler, J.B., and Cooney, T.G.: The pressure sore: pathophysiology and principles of management. Ann. Intern. Med., *94*:661–666, 1981.

Central Nervous Symptoms

1. Abramowicz, M. (Ed.): Choice of benzodiazepines. Med. Lett. Drugs Ther., *23*:41–43, 1981.
2. Black, P.: Brain metastasis: Current status and recommended guidelines for management. Neurosurgery, *5*:617–631, 1979.
3. Goldbert, R.J.: Management of depression in the patient with advanced cancer. J.A.M.A., *246*:373–376, 1981.
4. Gutin, P.: Corticosteroid therapy in patients with brain tumors. Natl. Cancer Inst. Monogr., *46*:151–156, 1977.
5. Hollister, L.E.: Tricyclic antidepressants. N. Engl. J. Med., *299*:1106–1109, 1168–1172, 1978.
6. Lieberman, A., et al.: Use of high dose corticosteroids in patients with inoperable brain tumors. J. Neurol. Neurosurg. Psychiatry, *40*:678–682, 1977.
7. McEvoy, J.P.: Organic brain syndromes. Ann. Intern. Med., *95*:212–220, 1981.
8. Posner, J.B.: Neurological complications of systemic cancer. Med. Clin. North Am., *63*:783–800, 1979.

Index

Page numbers in *italics* refer to illustrations; page numbers followed by "t" refer to tables.

dysfunctional response, 119, 120
guilt, 129, 134
loss of self-esteem, 132
pathologic grief, 130
regression, 122
suicidal ideation, 132
therapist and, role of, 119–136
therapy and, 123, 124
Fear, of abandonment, 15, 16
pain and, 78
Fecal impaction, 21, 219, 244–246
Fecal incontinence, 21, 232
Fever, 18
anti-inflammatory agents in, 19
from intrapleural therapy, 30
Fibrosis, as side effect of radiation
therapy, 69
Final decisions, 35
Flagyl, 252
Fleet's enemas. See *Enemas*
Fluid retention, extracellular, 32, 33
Fluocinolone, 249
Fluoxymesterone, 239, 252
Flurazepam, 255
Foley catheter, 248, 249
Food absorption and metabolism. See
Nutritional support
Fracture, 259
pathologic, 231
prophylaxis for, 231
Freamine, 146
Funeral practices, as social conceptions,
191
in other cultures, 190
in United States, 198
Fungating growths, 251
Fungizone, 240
Furosemide, 34

Gamma-aminobutyrate, 94. See also
Endorphin(s); Opiate receptors
Gastric carcinoma, radiation therapy and,
73
Gastric distention, 240, 241
Gastric irritation, 19, 241
Gastric outlet obstruction, 241
Gastrointestinal malignancies,
neuropathies in, 48
Gastrointestinal symptoms, 238
Gastrointestinal tract, dysfunction of, 17
obstruction of, 17
tumors of, 17
Gate control theory, of pain, 77, 83
Genetic alterations in cancer cells, 2, 3, 6,
7, 10
Genetic influence in tumor development,
11
Genetic instability in cancer cells, 2–4
Geural, 145

Gingivitis, 19
Glioma. See *Brain, malignancies of*
Globus pallidus, enkephalins in, 94
D-gluconic acid, 249
Glycerin suppository, 220
Goals, of terminal patients, 116
Granulex, 251
Grief, 128–131
as cultural phenomenon, 193, 195
pathologic, 130
symptoms of, 128, 129
Guillain-Barré syndrome, 48, 49. See also
*Neuromuscular disease(s),
neuropathy*
Guilt, and cancer, 113. See also *Family*
Gums, 19
Gyne-Lotrimin Vaginal Suppositories, 240

Habit disorders, hypnosis and, 86
Hair loss, 57
Haldol, 221, 242, 255, 256, 257
Haloperidol, 221, 242, 243, 255–257
Halotestin, 239, 252
Headache(s), 40
as sign of meningeal spread, 43
from intracranial tumor, 235
from neurologic dysfunction, 39, 40
radiation therapy and, 70
Helplessness, 24
Hematologic complications, 30
Hematologic malignancies, infection in, 27
Hematologic neoplasms, 30, 31
Heminevrin, 255
Hemiparesis, 39, 47
Hemoptysis, radiation therapy and, 73
Hemorrhage, 19, 73, 259
Hemorrhoids, 217
Hepatic aid in nutrition, 145
Hepatic dysfunction, 20
Hepatic enlargement, painful, 230, 241
Hepatic failure, 25
Hepatic glycogenolysis, 18
Hepatic infiltration, 17, 33
Hepatic vein thrombosis, 33
Heredity. See under *Genetic*
Heroin, 222, 223, 224
Herpes zoster, 237
Heterohypnosis, *85*
Hibiclens, 252
Hibitane, 249
Hiccoughs, 240, 241
High Pen Protein, 145
Hiprex, 249
Hodgkin's disease, 18, 19, 48, 49, 57
Home care, 30, 151–166
eligibility for, 154
hospice and, 153
of terminal patient, 151
reimbursement for, 152, 153, 155, 156
Horner's syndrome, 44, 45

conflict and, 212
prayer and, 206, 207
religious faith and, 116, 117, 210
spiritual needs of terminal patients and, 203, 204, 206
spiritual well-being and, 117, 203
Stadol, 105
Starvation, 138–139
Status epilepticus, 258
Steatorrhea, 20
Stelazine, 256, 257
Stiff neck, as sign of meningeal spread, 43
Stomach. See under *Gastric* and *Gastrointestinal*
Stomal care, 246, 251
Stool softeners, 21, 220, 244, 245
Substance P, gate theory of pain and, 99
Suffocation, 27, 30, 111
Suicide, 132, 175
Superior vena cava syndrome, 59
Supplemental oxygen, 29, 256
Supplements, nutritional, 143
Support, withdrawal of, legal issues and, 183
Suppositories, 245
Surgery, 16, 71, 230
Survivors, communication needs of, 130
Sustacal, 145
Swallowing problems, 19, 20, 240
Symptom control manual, 214–262
Synalar, 249

Tagamet, 20, 235, 240
Talwin, 104, 105, 224
Taste, 19
Tegretol, 237, 241, 258
Telfa, 251
Temaril, 250
Temgesic, 105
TENS (transcutaneous electrical nerve stimulation), 83, 233, 237
Terminal illness and terminal care,
adaptive defenses of patients and, 116
airway secretions and, 247, 257
as a family event, 120
legal issues of, 170
pain and, 223
perceived as punishment, 113
psychologic needs of patients and, 109, 117
restlessness and, 257
spiritual needs and, 203
transitions in families facing and, 119
Termination of care, legal issues and, 175, 186
Testicular cancer, 41
Tetracycline, 30
Tetrahydrocannabinol, 242, 243

Thiazides, 34
Thioridazine, 256, 257
Thirst, 22, 239
Thoracentesis, 29, 30
Thoracic problems in lung cancer, 29, 73
Thorazine, 221, 236, 241, 242, 247, 254, 255, 256, 257
Thrombocytopenia, 31, 47
Thrombotic endocarditis, 47
Thrush. See *Candida infection*
Tics, 237
Tofranil, 253
Tolerance, to opiates, 81, 105, 122
Toothache, 217
Topical anesthetics, 19,20
Tort law, medical care and, 168
Total enteral nutrition, 143, 144t
Total parenteral nutrition, 143, 146t
Toxic psychosis, 26
Toxoplasma, 46
Tranquilizers, 254, 256–257
Transcutaneous electrical nerve stimulation (TENS), 83, 233, 237
Transfusions, 28–30
Travasol, 146
Treatment decisions, 16, 117
Triamcinolone, 249
Tricyclic antidepressants, 239, 253
Trifluoperazine, 256, 257
Trigeminal nucleus, pain fibers in, 99
Trimeprazin, 250
Trimethoprim/sulfamethoxazole, 31, 248, 249
T-tube, 25
Tumor Angiogenesis Factor (TAF), 8
Tumor biology, 1–14
Tylenol, 224
Tylox, 224, 225

Unorthodox cancer treatment, 114
Urecholine, 31, 32, 248
Uremia, 18, 22, 35, 256
Ureter, obstruction in, 22
Urinary dysfunction and incontinence, 31, 42, 43, 248, 249. See also *Bladder*
Urinary tract infection, 26, 31, 33, 248
amoxicillin in, 248
asymptomatic bacteriuria and, 31

Valium, 237, 241, 247, 250, 254, 256, 257, 258
Valproic acid, 237, 258
Vascular disorders, 47
Veinamine, 146
Vena caval syndrome, radiation therapy and, 74
Venous obstruction and thrombosis, 32, 33
Veractil, 243, 244